RUNNING ON HOPE

POLICY T🌐 PRACTICE
Ethnographic Perspectives on Global Health Systems

SERIES EDITORS: Svea Closser, Emily Mendenhall, Judith Justice, & Peter J. Brown

Policy to Practice: Ethnographic Perspectives on Global Health Systems illustrates and provides critical perspectives on how global health policy becomes practice, and how critical scholarship can itself inform global public health policy. Policy to Practice provides a venue for relevant work from a variety of disciplines, including anthropology, sociology, history, political science, and critical public health.

Running On Hope

Female Community Health Labor in Rajasthan, India

SVEA CLOSSER AND SURENDRA SINGH SHEKHAWAT

VANDERBILT UNIVERSITY PRESS

Nashville, Tennessee

Library of Congress Cataloging-in-Publication Data

Names: Closser, Svea, 1978- author. | Shekhawat, Surendra Singh, author.
Title: Running on hope : female community health labor in Rajasthan, India
　/ Svea Closser and Surendra Singh Shekhawat.
Other titles: Policy to practice (Nashville, Tenn.) ; 4
Description: Nashville, Tennessee : Vanderbilt University Press, [2024] |
　Series: Policy to practice ; vol 4 | Includes bibliographical references
　and index.
Identifiers: LCCN 2024038185 (print) | LCCN 2024038186 (ebook) | ISBN
　9780826507631 (paperback) | ISBN 9780826507648 (hardcover) | ISBN
　9780826507655 (epub) | ISBN 9780826507662 (pdf)
Subjects: MESH: Community Health Workers | Women | Government Programs |
　India | Interview
Classification: LCC RA529 (print) | LCC RA529 (ebook) | NLM W 21.5 | DDC
　362.10954/4--dc23/eng/20250123
LC record available at https://lccn.loc.gov/2024038185
LC ebook record available at https://lccn.loc.gov/2024038186

For Rajasthan's ASHAs

CONTENTS

PEOPLE IN THIS BOOK

All names have been changed. The brief list here is for reference; we provide details on all of these people's experiences and perspectives in the main text.

Meena, whose story opens this book, has moved from rarely leaving the house, to being someone who helps community members around her navigate the health system, to working with ASHAs around her to unionize and advocate for greater benefits. Meena is an extraordinarily committed ASHA and union leader who feels betrayed both by the health system and the unions. She lives in a mid-size city in Rajasthan.

Bharti is the only ASHA in Gurha Sajjanpura that does not live with her extended family. Bharti has worked very hard to build a modest home, and to ensure that her two daughters, now both around twenty, are educated. She is an avid gardener.

Kavita is an ASHA who lives in a large home just outside of Gurha Sajjanpura, with many fields and cattle. She got a master's degree through correspondence courses. In addition to her work as an ASHA, she also works with her sister-in-law on embroidery and in the fields.

Anju also lives in a home just outside Gurha Sajjanpura, although hers is less well furnished than Kavita's. Anju has a nine-month-old baby. She zips around Gurha Sajjanpura on a motor scooter, veiled and confident.

Anita is a dynamic, charismatic ASHA who is a union leader. She worked under Shiv Partap for years, but then broke away in order to try becoming a union leader herself. Her vision is to form a union where ASHAs organize for themselves.

Shiv Partap is a union leader who holds a powerful bureaucratic position within the Rajsthani state government. He is sophisticated and strategic, artfully managing his many ties and political responsibilities.

Shafique is also a union leader. In addition to his ASHA union, he also has other unions, for example one for rickshaw drivers.

Seema is the most militant ASHA organizer we met, aiming to break away from established, male-led unions to lead one of her own. She and her friends have blocked cars, staged hunger strikes, and in their telling gotten into a physical altercation with the Minister of Women's Affairs.

Priya is an ASHA who became more involved in ASHA protests after COVID. She lives in a rural village outside Gurha Sajjanpura.

ACRONYMS

ANM: Auxiliary Nurse-Midwife. ANMs are female workers in India's health system, employed as permanent staff.

ASHA: Accredited Social Health Activist. ASHAs are an all-female cadre of Community Health Workers in India. The word *asha* also means "hope" in Hindi.

BA: Bachelor of Arts, a university degree.

BJP: Bharatiya Janata Party, a right-wing political party in India. The BJP is the party of populist leader Narendra Modi.

BMS: Bharatiya Mazdoor Sangh, a union affiliated with the BJP.

CHW: Community Health Worker.

CMHO: Chief Medical and Health Officer, a high-ranking official within the Indian health system.

FIR: First Information Report, a written document prepared by the police during a formal complaint of wrongdoing.

IAST: International Alphabet of Sanskrit Transliteration.

ICDS: Integrated Child and Development Services, an Indian program falling under the Department of Women and Child Development. Anganwadi Workers are the female village-level staff of ICDS; until 2022, ASHAs in Rajasthan worked for both ICDS and the Ministry of Health.

ICU: Intensive Care Unit, a part of the hospital.

IMF: International Monetary Fund.

MDRTB: Multi-Drug-Resistant Tuberculosis.

MGNREGA: Mahatma Gandhi National Rural Employment Guarantee Act.

NGO: Non-Governmental Organization.

SDGs: Sustainable Development Goals, a set of goals created by the United
Nations.

WHO: World Health Organization.

Preface

Our Collaboration

The work in this book is centered in a place we call Gurha Sajjanpura, a town of around ten thousand people in rural Rajasthan, an Indian state in a desert region in North India (fig. 1). Gurha Sajjanpura was once a center of power—there are imposing royal structures in town dating back to the 1400s—but they have fallen into disuse, and today the atmosphere is quiet. The town, easily traversed on foot, is made up of cement houses and a single sun-baked strip of stores connected by a jumble of roads just wide enough for a car. Outside of town, the landscape opens up and becomes greener; dirt roads traverse large fields dotted with the colorful figures of the women working in them. Many of Gurha Sajjanpura's men work in Rajasthan's capital city, Jaipur, a rapidly expanding desert megacity about an hour away.

Svea is a middle-aged white female anthropologist from the United States; Surendra is a young male anthropologist from Jaipur. We first met when Surendra was contracted by the Fulbright-Nehru program in India to help Svea get settled in Jaipur. That first meeting grew into a strong collaboration and deep friendship that now spans multiple research projects and life events over nearly a decade. We enjoy our collaboration greatly—we are both anthropology nerds, and in doing the work that led to this book we immersed ourselves in the process of refining research questions,

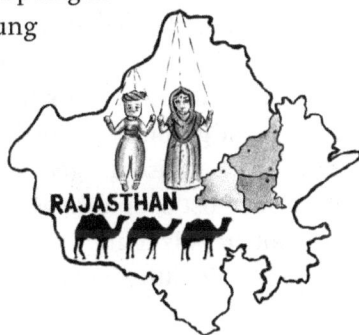

FIGURE 1.
Location of our fieldwork in Rajasthan, India. The ASHAs in this book lived and worked in the shaded area of the state. Illustration © Soniya Kanwar.

conducting interviews, and planning next steps. We found our complementary identities (male and female, younger and older, insider and outsider) helpful, both in conducting interviews and in thinking through our analysis.

We both stayed in Gurha Sajjanpura when we were conducting research, each of us with a different family; Surendra arranged these homestays and we paid the families we stayed with, although the atmosphere in the homes felt more like being family than renting. The houses were just around the block from each other. The structure of our days in Gurha Sajjanpura was quite consistent.

In the mornings, we would each get up in our respective houses, awakened by the bright light and intense heat of summer in Rajasthan. (Neither of the houses we stayed in, although lovely middle class homes by Gurha Sajjanpura standards, had air conditioning). We would each go downstairs and greet the families we were staying with; the daughters-in-law of the families would make us tea. As is normal in the system of gender segregation in Gurha Sajjanpura, which we will describe more in later chapters, Surendra rarely if ever saw these younger women's faces; Svea, as a woman, was free to participate in other women's worlds. In the mornings, Svea would sit with tea and biscuits in the common room of her house, chatting with the older couple who headed the household and playing with the kids, while the young women of the house strategically positioned themselves in the doorway so that Svea could see them and chat with them, but their father-in-law couldn't (as we discuss in Chapter 3, young married women limit the extent to which they are seen or heard by men in the household).

When it was time for breakfast, Svea would walk over to the house where Surendra was staying. This was a short walk of a block or two, on the dirt roads in this residential area of the village. There would always be people, cows, and sometimes goats or other animals on the street. Because Surendra had laid the groundwork for our work by making introductions throughout town, and because the gossip network in Gurha Sajjanpura was swift and effective, most people knew who we were and why we were there, and the atmosphere was friendly. As Svea walked, older women would sometimes engage her in little, friendly conversations.

Over breakfast, served in the public room of the house where Surendra was staying, we discussed the plan for the day. Surendra had usually made the necessary arrangements for our work in the evening of the day before, going around town and making phone calls asking people if they were willing to be interviewed, or if we could conduct participant observation. We would go over, together, what we were hoping to learn from the interviews or participant observation we would do that day, discussing between us lingering questions we were hoping to answer and our thoughts about what we had learned so far.

We conducted our interviews together, in Hindi, the national language of India. The local language in Gurha Sajjanpura is Dhundari, Surendra's native language, and a language that Svea doesn't speak. Most people in Gurha Sajjanpura were also fluent in Hindi; the ASHAs and other people who worked in government health posts had been formally educated in it since childhood. Conversations within the health post were already mostly in Hindi. So it felt natural to conduct interviews in Hindi, allowing Svea to participate. In the few cases where family members of ASHAs felt more comfortable speaking in Dhundari, Surendra conducted the interview.

We conducted our interviews wherever our interviewees preferred, which was usually at their place of work for ASHAs, and at their homes for family members. In very rare cases, interviewees preferred to come to us.

When we visited families at home, they always made us tea. The ethics review board in India had required us to get written informed consent from all of our respondents, and the first cup of tea usually was devoted to going over the written information sheet, answering questions about our study, and allowing our less literate respondents to get the informed consent sheet they were signing read by a more literate family member. We found that this process, which often took more than half an hour, was valuable in facilitating in-depth discussions about what we were doing and why. By the time the interview began, we were often on the second cup of tea, and our interviewees were well informed about what kind of information we were looking for and often quite invested in helping us with our work. This extended informed consent process helped lay the groundwork for talking in an open, conversational way.

We conducted our interviews collaboratively, each of us asking questions whenever one came to mind. We did this because it worked well; our interview styles are similar, and we were on the same page about what we wanted out of our interviews. We both feel that often, the other person would ask the perfect follow-up question of our interviewee, one that we ourselves had not quite formulated. Sometimes, when Svea tripped over her words in Hindi, Surendra would clarify what she was trying to ask.

We also conducted participant observation collaboratively. Svea does not blend in in rural Rajasthan, so in cases where some people at the events we were observing did not already know who we were, it was natural as well as ethical for us to introduce ourselves and explain our project. This was made easier by the fact that ASHAs who knew us were almost always present when we did participant observation, so we were never total strangers. We explained what we were doing, and the kinds of notes we would be taking. Generally speaking, people in health care settings were somewhat mildly interested but overall not very bothered by our presence; we had permission letters from state-level authorities allowing us to do the work, and observers of various types were fairly common in the Rajasthani health system. In union settings, ASHAs were generally quite pleased that we were there, as they were hoping for more visibility for their efforts and they saw our documentation as contributing to that.

We both participated in the same events, but we took independent jottings throughout the day. Most of the interactions we were observing during participant observation in health centers and union events took place in Hindi. The interactions between ASHAs and the community members they served, however, were mostly in Dhundari, so Surendra could pick up much more of what was happening in those interactions.

After conducting participant observation, in the evening or the next morning, we would write fieldnotes collaboratively from the jottings each of us had taken. We would meet in a public room in one of the houses where we were staying, and go over what we had learned. We discussed the events we had witnessed, putting together details of what we had seen from the jottings each of us had taken in our notebooks. Svea typed the more formal fieldnotes up in English on her computer as we talked, drawing details from the notes both of us had taken.

We analyzed the material later, when Svea was back at home in Baltimore, in the United States, and Surendra was at home in Jaipur, the capital of Rajasthan. During the long hours of COVID lockdowns, Surendra listened to the recordings of our interviews and transcribed them in Hindi in notebooks. Then, in hours of Zoom and WhatsApp calls, in the morning for Svea and in the evening for Surendra, we worked through the Hindi transcripts together to translate them into English. Svea typed up those English transcripts as we worked. In some cases, when English didn't quite capture the meaning, we kept the original Hindi, written out in Roman characters.

In this book, we have sometimes included material in Hindi (along with English translations), mostly in places where the words in English were not as poetic or resonant as what our interviewees actually said to us. For the transliterated Hindi, we used International Alphabet of Sanskrit

Transliteration (IAST) conventions, except in places where there is a more commonly used spelling of a Hindi word in roman characters (for example, for the title of a village leader, we used the common spelling of *sarpanch* rather than the IAST spelling *sarpañca).* We hope this makes the book come alive a bit more for our Hindi-speaking readers.

Next, over Zoom and WhatsApp calls, we discussed the themes we wanted to write about—something that was clear to us at this point due to our collaborative, careful work with both our fieldnotes and our transcripts, as well as what by now had become personal connections to the ASHAs involved in our project. Although we did not formally code our material, Surendra looked over all of the interviews and transcripts again, highlighting material that was particularly useful for each of the themes we were covering. Together, we discussed which ASHAs would be featured as main characters in the book.

Once we agreed on the material that we thought was essential for the book, Svea put all of the vignettes and the important ideas on index cards, and arranged those cards into chapters. She then typed up the resulting outline, and both of us discussed, refined, and improved it.

Svea next wrote up each chapter from the materials we had put together. As she wrote, she aimed for accessibility. We wanted this book to be engaging for both policymakers and students, two of our primary audiences for this book.

Anthropological theory has informed the thinking in this book profoundly. The many articles we cite in the footnotes of this book are great resources for people interested in more theoretical background on many of the dynamics we describe. In the conclusion, we offer a few theoretical observations for other anthropologists. But for the most part, aware that much anthropological work can be unreadable to those working in global public health, we tried not to have the narrative get too bogged down in theory. The written material in this book focuses on the experiences of the ASHAs we knew.

We went over each draft chapter together, reading aloud, on more Zoom and WhatsApp calls, discussing the material and our analysis of the material. Svea made edits as we worked. The resulting book is deeply and thoroughly a collaborative project, to the point that it is impossible for us to pinpoint whose contributions are whose. All of the thinking here was developed together, and neither of us could have done the work or made the arguments in this book alone.

We think that the nature of our collaboration shows how misleading it can be to use the term "research assistant," a dismissive term too often used by American-trained anthropologists for their very skilled South Asian collaborators. We recently heard the Indian research assistant of a prominent American anthropologist described as her "secret weapon"—which for us raised the question: why was this collaborator a secret?

Part of the answer to this question is in the structure of American anthropology, which, wedded to the "lone wolf" ideal, may reward young anthropologists with jobs and tenure only if they write as if they conducted research alone. In fact, of course, few anthropologists get very far without a lot of friends and a lot of mentoring at their field site—this is true even if they do their fieldwork in the country where they grew up. The danger is that the myth of the lone wolf can blind American-trained anthropologists to the extent of the support they receive: it can lead them to refer to their teachers as their "assistants," and to believe that the language reflects the reality.

The neocolonial aspects of the foreign "researcher" and the local "research assistant" are perhaps too obvious to belabor here, except to say that a change in this language is long overdue. Two other ethnographers of Rajasthan, Ann Gold and Bhoju Ram Gujar, coauthored a book in 2002.[1] This step is obviously appropriate in many anthropological collaborations; it should not still be so rare.

CHAPTER 1

Call Whenever You Need Me

Rajasthan's Community Health Workers

A public hospital in rural Rajasthan, India was very busy on a sweltering summer day in 2018. Although a storm was gathering, in the crowded courtyard in front of the building, two lines of people—one for women, one for men—jostled to get the entry tickets they would need to get care.

The two of us looked around for Meena. Meena was an ASHA, or Accredited Social Health Activist, a Community Health Worker in India's government health system. We had been following her life and story.

Meena finally arrived, an hour later than expected, rushing and carrying a bag of paperwork, lighting up and greeting us warmly when she saw us. She was a woman of around thirty, perfectly turned out as always, today in a vibrant navy and pink sari and a richly colored blue sari blouse. We followed her inside through the hospital, the wards overflowing with multiple people on beds packing the hallways. She was late, she explained, because she had been at the hospital all night helping to deliver a baby. Did we want to come with her while she checked on the mother?

The delivery ward was so crowded that we could barely make our way in. Meena led us to a bed near the door, where a weary, ecstatic new mother pulled up some covers to reveal a sleeping newborn. The baby was tiny and perfect: the mother, the father, the baby's toddler brother, and the thrilled grandmother warmly pulled both Meena and her two anthropologists into their circle of elation and joy.

The baby was a girl, the grandmother explained, laying her arm over Svea's. Gesturing to the mother, she said, "Everything is great now. A brother and a sister, now we are free from worry!"

Then the grandmother gushed, "Meena is doing everything. Back in the old days, it was the mother and father who cared for their child. And now what has happened, it's the ASHAs who do everything. *They* take care of the children!"

Meena laughed and shook her head, saying that that was the truth. ASHAs had a huge amount of responsibility.

"They Called Me, and I Came"

Meena's first order of business this morning—one of the most important parts of her job—was to start preparing the mother's paperwork. The Rajasthani government had recently started an incentive program, called Mukhyamantree Rājśrī Yojanā (more or less literally translated, the Prime Minister's Brilliant Idea), designed to narrow the survival and education gaps between boy and girl children in a setting of severe gender inequality. Mothers received cash incentives when they gave birth to a female child in a health facility, when they vaccinated their daughter, when the daughter enrolled in school, and when the daughter completed secondary education. (To try to reduce the preferential treatment often given to boys, these incentives were only for daughters; this incentive program paralleled a global enthusiasm for investment in girls as a way to produce economic gains).[1]

There was paperwork for these incentives for the family; there was paperwork for Meena's documentation that she had helped the family with the delivery. This was only a small sliver of the paperwork that made up much of Meena's job, documenting (among many other things) child weights, immunization status, antenatal care visits, tuberculosis patient medication compliance, what kinds of family planning people were using, and even whether families had installed gutters on the roof of their homes. She did all of this for every family in her catchment area, around a thousand people. The data Meena generated through this voluminous, labor-intensive paperwork tied her invisibly to government health administrators at district, state, and national levels, and to a large network of global health policymakers using that data to evaluate programs and make decisions.[2]

None of the people in the small family before us was literate; they had moved to Meena's neighborhood only two years ago, when their home in the city of Jaipur, a sprawling desert metropolis that is the capital of Rajasthan, was destroyed by the government because it was built on land not zoned for residential use. They badly needed the economic assistance these government incentives would provide. But to get them, the mother needed two different ID cards and a bank account—and she had none of these things. Meena would help her navigate the paperwork and the bureaucracy to get them, bringing her forms, collecting documents, and ferrying them to the health center and the bank.

As payment for her efforts in helping this family—going with them to the hospital, staying up all night, checking in on the family, completing piles of paperwork—Meena would receive 300 rupees (about US $5). It was not enough, she commented to us, for many hours of work and missing a night of sleep.

At 2:30 a.m. that morning, this woman's family had called Meena. She got up, called the ambulance, met the ambulance, and directed them to the woman's house. Meena brought them all to the hospital, helping the woman navigate the check-in and paperwork; moving her through the hospital to the maternity ward; and acting as a mediator and guide between the mother and the hospital staff. At 6 a.m. the baby was born; Meena stayed until seven. Then Meena went home, made up her children's lunches for the day, and brought her children to school. After that, she showered, went to the local child-care center where she also had responsibilities as an ASHA, and now was back at the hospital. She had barely slept. But when we left the delivery room, Meena explained to us:

> Those people just came here from Jaipur two years ago. People who've been around for a while, they've been through the process of delivering a baby, they have some experience, so they know where to go, what they need to do. But this family, they didn't know any of that. The poor woman was so frightened. She asked me to help. I told her, whenever you need me, you can call. And this morning at 2:30 a.m., she called.
>
> The thing is, when you are there for people, then you build trust. It means something to them: they called me, and I came. That's why people in my area trust me more than anyone else in the health system. This morning, when I got back home from the hospital, a woman was waiting for me at my house. I brought her with me to the hospital, and showed her the line to get her entry ticket. I'll help her through the hospital. You know, she believes in me.

Meena had been an ASHA for more than ten years; she had built up trust with people in her community over time. The ASHA title (pronounced "ah-sha") reads as an acronym, but it was much more than an acronym to Meena and everyone else in the health system in Gurja Sajjanpura. The word *asha* in Hindi means "hope," and ASHAs were nearly universally seen as critical links between the health system and the people that system aimed to serve.

"My Family, They Tell Me to Quit"

At first, the job had been a real challenge. When Meena started her work, she had been a young mother with two toddlers. At the time, the salary was Rs 500 (around $10) per month. Meena had moved to this town only after her marriage. Following the conventions of young married Hindu women in Rajasthan, at that time she rarely left the house, and did so only veiled. She knew little of the world outside her walls. She explained:

> My husband had forbidden me to take the job: "You're going to abandon the children for $10 a month?"
>
> But my mother-in-law said, "Everything is so expensive these days, and this way she'll be standing on her own two feet. She'll take care of her own family herself." Then my husband had to go along. My mother-in-law said, "I'll take care of the children, you go." My mother- and father-in-law have experienced great poverty, so they understood the value of a job.
>
> But at the beginning, it was so difficult! At the beginning, they told us that each day, we had to do a survey of ten households. And my catchment area was huge. I didn't know anything! If I ever left the house, my mother-in-law used to make sure that not even my teeth were showing from under my sari. She would scold me: "Your teeth are showing! Your chin is showing! The neighbors are watching!" Think of it, in that situation how would I go out and do a door-to-door survey?
>
> But my father-in-law, he was a pandit [priest]. Everyone knew me as the pandit's daughter-in-law. He went with me when I went door to door. He supported me. He told everyone, "This is my daughter-in-law, and she just started work as an ASHA. Whatever you need, tell her and she'll get it for you."

Meena had grown into the job. After almost ten years of work, she now did it easily on her own. But the hours could be brutal, and the pay was awful. She and her family were both ambivalent, she explained:

> Sometimes I get stressed about all the work, and my family, they tell me to quit. But the thing is, I have worked so hard to get to know all those people, and even if I quit they'll still come to me asking for help! I won't be able to say no.

And then, I think, what am I getting out of this work? I mean, in terms of living a good life. Whatever heartbreak I have at home, whatever pain and problem I am facing, I forget it all, when I work with these people.

In the past few years my father died. My brother had kidney disease, he died too. When I'm at work, I'm not thinking about those things. Helping others, I forget.

And the people I've met, they've become family. I don't dwell on my sadness. So that's why I tell myself: I've made so many friends, I've learned so many things. And I have left the house and gotten to know the wider world.

Meena had gotten to know this world better than many of her male relatives. When her brother fell ill, she was the one who took him to a faraway city and guided him through the hospital system. And at home, she had taken on much of the work running errands and visiting relatives—something she never would have done before.

Yet despite her expanded freedom, Meena's job remained stressful and the pay very low. Every ASHA in Gurha Sajjanpura commented to us that their pay was low. Teachers, they pointed out, could earn 50,000 rupees a month (about $700). But between their base salary of 2,500 rupees and the incentive-based payments they got, most of Gurja Sajjanpura's ASHAs averaged around Rs 6,000 (about $80) per month. It was, we heard repeatedly, "nothing."

Meena, like the other ASHAs she worked with, waited for the day when their job might become a "permanent" government position, one with minimum wage pay and benefits. Because they worked so hard and provided so much, they hoped that the government would recognize those contributions with job security. They were, Meena explained, "running on hope."

Health by the People

India's 900,000 ASHAs make up the largest Community Health Worker (CHW) program in the world. CHWs are the backbone of the health systems in contexts like India, where there are not enough doctors and nurses in rural areas to cover the population with basic health services. The CHW model is common worldwide; Ethiopia's Health Extension Worker program, as just one of many examples, also employs local women to provide essential health services in remote areas and underserved urban settings alike. CHWs bridge the social and service delivery gaps between communities and health systems, and they have long been held up as the embodiment of community participation and empowerment in health.

Long before the ASHA program, India was home to a pioneering Community Health Worker program. In 1970, Rajanikant and Mabelle Arole founded the Jamkhed Comprehensive Rural Health Project in the state of Maharashtra. The Aroles were medical doctors who had been stationed at a rural hospital, but they soon found that their efforts as physicians were not addressing the root causes of illness. The underlying causes of poor health, from inadequate nutrition to poor sanitation, would continue to make people sick, and their efforts at curative care were not addressing these issues. They explained:

> After four years of service we recognized that 70 percent of illnesses were preventable and large numbers of patients "cured" in the hospital were going back to the same environment and later returning to the hospital for the same sort of episode of illness. This repetitive pattern of simple preventable illnesses could not be changed by the hospital even though it was situated in the heart of the rural area. Since a traditional curative-oriented hospital system does not penetrate the communities and does not see patients as a part of a community in relation to the environment they live in, it fails to meet the total needs of the community.[3]

The Aroles centered their project around marginalized women, teaching illiterate widows and *Dalits* (a low-caste group in India) to provide basic health services and health education.[4] For example, they reached out to the families of underweight children, providing supplemental nutrition support. They encouraged immunization and referred mothers who had danger signs during pregnancy. These female Community Health Workers were extraordinarily effective. In just five years, the infant mortality rate was cut by two thirds, and both antenatal care coverage and immunization rates went from near zero to more than eighty percent.[5]

The project was enormously influential at a global level, not only for its effectiveness, but for its ethos. In his landmark book *Health by the People*, published by the World Health Organization in 1975, Kenneth Newell highlighted the Jamkhed project, commenting that it was not enough to think of health in terms of disease burden, rates of child stunting, and maternal deaths. Instead, Newell argued, health planners should focus on "such qualities as hope, human dignity, a capacity for improvement and change, organization and responsibility, and mastery over one's own fate."[6]

The Jamkhed project, along with other pioneering CHW programs in South Africa, Guatemala, and China, shaped an emerging vision of what was being called Primary Health Care.[7] Throughout the 1970s, there was growing momentum for community-based provision of comprehensive health services globally. In part, this was a philosophical movement away from single-disease programs targeting malaria and smallpox, and toward a vision of health care provision where everyone could access basic health services, provided conveniently and affordably, as a basic health right.[8]

This culminated in the landmark Alma-Ata conference in 1978. The Alma-Ata Declaration articulated a vision of the future in which communities actively participated in the provision of proven, socially acceptable health care.[9] The Alma-Ata document passionately argued against health inequality; stated that health was a "fundamental human right;" argued for health provided in accessible ways by and for communities; and emphasized that nutrition, education, and housing were all health issues.[10] It was a model rooted in a vision of social justice, and Community Health Workers were a core part of that vision.

Lackey or Liberator?

Even as momentum grew for the lofty ideals of Alma-Ata, however, some observers urged caution. The lofty ideals of community-based Primary Health Care are hard to achieve, and not always appealing to those in power. In the mid-1970s, David Werner, author of *Where There Is No Doctor*, visited forty rural health projects in nine Latin American countries. "We were inspired by some of the things we saw," he wrote of the projects' deployment of CHWs, "and profoundly disturbed by others. While in some of the projects we visited people were in fact regarded as a resource to control disease, in others we had a sickening impression that disease was being used as a resource to control people."[11]

Werner was concerned that Community Health Workers were being managed in a deeply problematic way by the programs that employed them— that they were, in his words, made to be lackeys rather than liberators. He continued:

> We find, in certain programs, a different breed of village health worker is being moulded—one who is taught a pathetically limited range of skills, who is trained not to think but to follow a list of very specific instructions or "norms,"

who has a neat uniform and a handsome diploma, who works in a standard-ized cement-block health post, and who is subject to restrictive supervision and rigidly predefined limitations. Such a health worker has a limited impact on the health and even less on the growth of the community. He, or more usu-ally she, spends a great deal of time filling out forms.[12]

If, as in the conception that underlies the tenets of Alma-Ata, health is most powerfully shaped by social justice—access to land, to food, to clean water, to communities' ability to determine their own priorities, including health priorities—then CHWs should be advocates for social justice and com-munity health. They should see equitable distribution of food as much as their priority as the provision of medicine. Yet such a vision of CHWs is often not particularly appealing to those in power—the policymakers and doctors that have the most influence in shaping CHW programs. These actors tend to want CHWs to serve and assist them, not to upend existing hierarchies.

In practice, CHW programs are often designed so that CHWs are not activists, but low-level laborers carrying out the tasks dictated to them from above. Often, CHWs around the world are disempowered staff at the bot-tom of health bureaucracies, facing severe restrictions on their ability to advocate for themselves or for the needs of their communities. They are frequently given strict orders on how to work, and little latitude to raise up health issues that are priorities for community members. Thus, there are long-standing tensions between "bottom-up" and "top-down" approaches to CHW work.[13] The scholar Kerry Scott, a close observer of the ASHA program in India, summarizes these "debates and tensions" (Table 1). They exem-plify the difference between the "liberator" model, envisioned in places like Alma-Ata, and the "lackey" model, embodied by Werner's description of the form-filling and heavily supervised health worker. These tensions run to the heart of CHW programs, including the ASHA program.

"Every Responsibility Falls on the ASHA"

It was time for the biweekly ASHA meeting at the hospital where Meena worked. Fifteen or twenty ASHAs sat on the floor, on a large carpet spread out in the hallway. We took a seat near Meena on the floor.

Chairs were lined up in front of the carpet. A male supervisor sat in one of them, flanked by the male computer operator and the female Auxiliary

Table 1. Kerry Scott's Debates and Tensions in CHW Programs

LIBERATOR	LACKEY
Self-motivated	Self-interested
Volunteer	Employee
Activist	Extender
Of and for the community	Of and for the health system
Empowered	Exploited

Source: Marta Schaaf et al., "Report on the 'Think-in' on Community Health Worker Voice, Power, and Citizens' Right to Health" (Accountability Research Center, January 2018), 10.

Nurse-Midwife (ANM), looking down on the group of ASHAs. The hospital's main doctor, a man, joined them on the chairs a little late.

The male supervisor started the meeting by saying sternly, "This meeting won't be over until all of your lists are verified. There's no excuse for having the registers being anything other than 100 percent correct. I've explained this to you before; I shouldn't have to tell you again."

The ASHAs' response to this opening salvo was heated. The register in question, they explained, was the responsibility of the Auxiliary Nurse-Midwife, and they should not have been tasked with it. "You're forcing us to do other people's work," one ASHA called out.

The vehemence of the response was not a matter of a single register. The ASHAs were frequently tasked with the work of their supervisors. An ASHA next to Svea leant over her notebook, where she was jotting fieldnotes. "Write this: We're doing the ANM's work. We're doing the *panchayat*'s work. Why should we do all of that?"

Several ASHAs in the room had taken it upon themselves to travel hours to Jaipur, the state capital, to meet with Ministry of Health officials. They met, they said, with the Chief Medical and Health Officer (CMHO), a high ranking official. "We won't fill the register, it's not our job," another ASHA called out. "The CMHO in Jaipur *clearly* told us not to."

In the midst of the meeting, the lights went out. It was pouring outside, and thunder rumbled. This fit the mood of the meeting, which was tumultuous, an argument between those on the chairs and those on the floor. The ASHAs were unruly and vocal. Half of them had let their saris slip off their heads. The more powerful people in the room, sitting on chairs, clapped their hands in the hope of restoring order. The Auxiliary Nurse-Midwife looked seriously displeased.

The ASHAs' refusal to do this paperwork—paperwork which was, in fact, not their responsibility—had had negative repercussions for the doctor and the hospital management, who had been called out at state meetings for not having proper documentation. They were redoubling pressure on the ASHAs in hopes of getting them to do it. It wasn't really working.

Meena was the most vocal of all the ASHAs at the meeting. She spoke back to the supervisor clearly and firmly, in a steady voice. But as she did so, her hand worried at her purse handle, nervously fingering the straps even as she strongly stated the ASHAs' case. She rocked just a little. She was nervous and simmering mad.

Later, a few ASHAs explained to us that their anger was rooted in the severe discrepancy between the work they do and the pay they get. "Everyone is our supervisor," they said. "Everyone dumps their work on us."

Meena was more sanguine: "There are only two Auxiliary Nurse-Midwives—how much work can they do? They get assigned the night shift. And they are forced to do the work of *their* supervisors, too. We need to have a good rhythm, good relations. Then the work will keep going."

Still, she commented, it wasn't fair: "We are the ones that fill out *every* field report. If there's any work that involves getting up from the desk, it becomes the ASHA's responsibility. And the manual labor: last night I stayed late emptying coolers and water tanks."

Another ASHA added, "If there's a dengue patient, a malaria patient, it's the ASHA who will follow up and do the paperwork. And look for more cases. Every responsibility falls on the ASHA, but the ASHAs are paid nothing."

No Love Without Fear

In the years after Alma-Ata, new CHW programs were founded across the world. India initiated a huge CHW program in the late 1970s, aiming for one worker for every one thousand people. The aim was to put "people's health in people's hands."[14] This move drew on a long history of support for CHWs in India, dating back to the freedom movement of the 1940s. Members of the freedom movement envisioned a community-based health system that would democratize knowledge; they wrote that CHWs should be a "cornerstone" of this system.[15]

Yet the massive CHW program scaled up in the 1970s faced challenges. One challenge—shared by CHW programs across the world—was opposition from doctors, who moved to protect their turf.[16] Anthropologist Mark Nichter observed that doctors in Indian health posts tended to "underplay the skills of field staff and jealously guard medical supplies for symbolic as well as economic reasons."[17]

Doctors wanted CHWs to be underlings under *their* control, not community control. In Werner's terms, they wanted lackeys, not liberators. In one example, researcher Rushikesh Maru noted in 1980 that although on paper, CHWs were to be controlled by the community, health staff had wrested control of CHW activities back. When Maru asked health post officials in India about CHWs, they insisted that top-down control of CHW activities was essential. "Control is a must because people are dishonest," one health post official told him. Another, arguing for intimidation tactics in managing CHWs, quipped, "There is no love without fear." Maru concluded that the Indian health bureaucracy was able to successfully resist "any new innovation which undermines its power to command and punish."[18]

The CHWs of the 1970s and early 1980s, who were mostly men, received a small stipend and a supply of medicines, but did not get a salary or benefits.[19] But once CHWs were treated as underlings by the health system, they began to feel that they deserved a wage.[20] It proved very difficult to maintain momentum over many years in a program that relied on workers that were paid very little. As CHWs began striking to demand fair wages, the government phased out the program.[21]

These developments in India mirrored the trajectory of many other CHW programs globally. Many programs fizzled out after a brief lifespan, in large part because training and remunerating huge cadres of CHWs was perceived to be too expensive. Structural Adjustment Programs implemented by the International Monetary Fund (IMF) in the 1980s and 1990s required the privatization of many industries, emptying government health system budgets. They pushed away from a model of health care as a social good and toward the privatization and commodification of health care.[22] Health systems, drained of money by neoliberal policies including these Structural Adjustment Programs, simply could not afford large scale salaried CHW initiatives.[23]

Thus, in the 1980s and 1990s, international enthusiasm for and attention to Primary Health Care and CHW programs waned. International initiatives, in India and elsewhere, overwhelmingly focused on "vertical" programs aimed at a few select diseases and delivered in a targeted way, not the broad-scale goals of Primary Health Care.[24]

However, in the 2000s and 2010s, CHW programs saw a global resurgence, paralleling the huge increases in funding and attention given to global public health in the wake of the HIV/AIDS pandemic. In the context of a global shortage of doctors and nurses, CHWs were seen as a way to get essential health services to those most in need. In this new environment, CHW programs were pitched as cost-*saving* strategies.[25] This framing of CHWs as a cost-effective solution to health labor shortages has far-reaching implications.

Power and Political Economy in Health Systems

Since the field of medical anthropology was born in the 1970s, medical anthropologists have explored the social organization, power relations, and politics of health systems. Ethnographers have worked to understand the lives and worlds of policymakers and health staff, as points of entry into the power structures that run through the global health enterprise. The tradition of studying health systems from the *inside* dates back to the pioneering work of Judith Justice, whose classic book *Policies, Plans and People* explored, among other things, the role of the "peon" in the Nepali health system. Officially the person tasked with getting tea for the doctor, peons were often preferred providers at rural health posts because they were knowledgeable, respectful, and connected to the communities they served.[26]

Fifteen years ago, the Critical Anthropology of Global Health (CAGH) Interest Group, part of the Society for Medical Anthropology, articulated a "health systems perspective" as a core anthropological contribution to global public health, pointing out that anthropologists could provide important insights on the economies, politics, and governance of health systems.[27] More recently, Katerini Storeng and Arima Mishra have shown that ethnographic work can illuminate health systems "in historical, political, and social perspective."[28] Karina Kielmann has noted that anthropological work can provide an "in-depth, rich, and nuanced analysis of the relationship between power, knowledge, and practice in health systems."[29] This book fits securely in that tradition.

Within this body of work, there is a growing literature on *healers* working within under-resourced government health systems.[30] And the anthropological literature on Community Health Workers is particularly strong. There are several resounding themes within this body of work.

Volunteer or Exploited Worker?

Many CHWs across the world are described as volunteers. ASHA work pays far less than minimum wage, on the legal grounds that it the work is "voluntary." The term volunteer in these contexts is slippery and often misleading: many volunteer CHWs globally get per diems or payments of some type that they consider pay—albeit awful pay.[31] Anthropologists have argued that the extremely low pay in most CHW programs leads to exploitative conductions in a wide variety of contexts.[32] Many "volunteer" CHWs are volunteers only in the sense that their often irregular remuneration is less than minimum wage.

Necessity is the driving force for low-paid or unpaid labor in many cases—a Community Health Worker force covering the population of even a small country will be a large number of people, and many Ministries of Health simply do not have money for a living wage for that many people in their budgets.[33] There are around one million ASHAs in India; even small changes in remuneration, multiplied by a million, add up to serious money very quickly. Paying CHWs the minimum amount required to get them to work means saving as much money as possible for other critical needs of the health system, such as lifesaving basic medications for impoverished patients.

Yet, this extremely low pay has profound consequences for CHWs. Anthropological work has shown that CHWs across contexts live in poverty.[34] CHWs across the world have taken up community health work as one income generating tactic among many, "volunteering" as a subsistence strategy in the hope that it will build social connections and one day result in a stable job.[35] Further, many CHWs hope—a hope that goes unfulfilled in most cases— that low-paid work as a CHW might eventually lead to a more stable job in the health system, or to political connections that would benefit them.[36]

CHW "volunteerism" has been justified by global health officials with a range of discursive strategies, the most common of which being that volunteers are intrinsically motivated, and that pay would interfere with intrinsic motivation.[37] Anthropologists have been quick to point out that those arguments are rarely applied to positions occupied by doctors, policymakers, or other high-status individuals.[38]

Many CHWs, of course, do find joy and meaning in their work.[39] A large body of anthropological work has shown that the desire to serve others coexists with an acute need for money in the motivations of many CHWs across the world.[40]

Women: the "Superior CHWs"

The new CHW programs of the 2000s and 2010s, which include India's ASHA program, are overwhelmingly made up of women. Out of the estimated five million CHWs serving their communities across the world, there are approximately twice as many female CHWs as there are male.[41] These women are tasked with providing care and saving lives at the front lines of often weak and unreliable health systems. As a recent World Health Organization (WHO) report put it, health services across the world are delivered by women—women who are managed by men.[42]

One reason for this is that women are often socially well positioned for the maternal and child health work that is central to many CHW programs. In Rajasthan, as in many other communities in South Asia, unrelated men are not always granted access to new mothers and newborn babies, but female CHWs are free to meet them. As we describe in this book, rural Rajsthani households have strict geographies of gender segregation, and in most households men simply could not do the kind of work that Meena does.

There are ideological reasons as well. Women are frequently idealized as caring and connected to their communities. For example, a Columbia University report promoting CHW programs said that women "often are superior CHWs" compared to men, due, in part, to "their attachment to the community, and their less common use of alcohol in evenings."[43] These constructions of female commitment and virtue echo others throughout global health and development programs, where women are portrayed as people whose gender makes them more caring, more giving, and more moral.[44] There are several deep issues with these narratives, which can function to mask and enable relationships of exploitation and domination.[45]

Often rhetoric around care posits caring as if it is something that an *individual* does, whereas care actually occurs in relationships.[46] "It makes little sense to think of individuals as if they were Robinson Crusoe, all alone, making decisions," scholar Joan Tronto writes.[47] Instead, caring happens in relationship with others, and carers themselves need support and care. As the stories in this book show, this is definitely true for CHWs.

Also, narratives of certain groups of people as caring or altruistic are almost always tied up in relations of power. Some groups of people—usually more powerful people—get a societal "pass" out of being caring or altruistic, because they are doing other things (making money, governing countries) that are presumably more important. At the same time, people constructed as being particularly caring are often assumed to be unconcerned with things like stable incomes, safe living environments, or gaining power—whether or not this is actually the case.[48]

Conceptualizing community health work as something that altruistic women do for their neighbors also can hide recognition that the work is often dangerous. Frontline health workers put their bodies in dangerous situations—exposing themselves to infection, and dealing with the emotional labor of interacting with a wide range of community members, including those who may not want the services they are providing.[49] Many CHWs are exposed to violence.[50] And sexual harassment and violence, both from supervisors and community members, can be common.[51]

Narratives of female virtue and giving, which circulate in centers of global health power across the world, can eclipse the fact that CHWs are not saints but humans—humans who usually desire fair pay and good working conditions.[52] Obscured by the rhetoric about female morality, but frequently behind the choice to deploy women, is the fact that men often will not work for the low or nonexistent pay offered CHWs. Women, who have fewer employment opportunities and a narrower radius of movement in many social contexts including Rajasthan, are often more willing to accept a very low wage—a set of dynamics that we will describe in detail in this book.[53] The Columbia report quoted earlier hints at this, saying that women "are less likely to abandon their posts as CHWs for better opportunities."[54]

Many countries besides India, including Nepal and Ethiopia, transitioned their volunteer CHW programs from male to female workers in the last fifty years; these transitions were influenced in part by stringent demands by male CHWs for more payment.[55] Someone with familiarity with internal discussions in India told us that women were favored as ASHAs in part because of the Indian government's previous experience with male CHWs; women were seen as less likely to be vocal or to unionize.

The Birth of the ASHA Program

The Mitanin program, started in the Indian state of Chhattisgarh in 2002, is a paradigmatic example of volunteer, community-engaged CHWs. Female CHWs called Mitanins were selected by their communities, through a facilitated process that elevated "weaker voices" and limited the power of local elites.[56] Conceptualized as "state-initiated community activism," the program was run and supported by the State Health Resource Center, an entity that brought together civil society, health experts, and government officials.[57]

Mitanins were trained as health activists, for example taking action to make sure that families who were food insecure were getting the government entitlements that were due them. In this program, the volunteer model seems to have worked very well. In part, this may have been because there was a rationale for volunteerism that did not rely particularly heavily on constructions of women as inherently virtuous. Instead, the volunteer nature of the program was a calculated move to disrupt the usual power dynamics. The rationale was that if Mitanins were paid employees at the lowest level of the government health system, they were likely to be answerable to the system, not the community.[58] Still, even this program eventually gave incentives to Mitanins for tasks that the state wanted accomplished— incentives that some observers felt were part of a process of pulling Mitanins away from activist work and into the top-down command structure of local elites.[59]

Even so, the program had some notable successes. Mitanins took on local elites, even identifying corruption within the health system. They protected themselves by forming alliances, including a state-wide network of Mitanins with powerful support at the state level.[60]

The success of the Mitanin program influenced the nascent ASHA program. In the mid-2000s, the Indian government created the ambitious National Rural Health Mission, a program aiming to expand effective health services to India's vast rural population. The ASHA was a key part of the National Rural Health Mission's design.

The Mitanin program was an inspiration and a model to those designing the ASHA program—up to a point. When the Mitanin model was taken up by powerful donors and national policymakers in Delhi, someone familiar with the process told us, "they took some of the convenient components"— meaning the parts palatable to those in power—"and left out some of the less convenient components."

While Mitanins had been given job security (albeit low-paid or unpaid job security), ASHAs would not be so secure. The neoliberal atmosphere that surrounded the creation of the National Rural Health Mission was one in which contractual, temporary work was increasingly the norm globally. At that time—and now—there was little or no appetite in donor organizations for the recurring costs involved in hiring large cadres of health workers.[61] Nor were governments always enthusiastic about such investments.

Two people familiar with the negotiations of the early ASHA program told us independently that the government was unwilling to provide these new workers with paid employment.

The incentive structure of the ASHA program evolved in a way that reflected broader trends in the CHW resurgence of the early 2000s. It was agreed that the ASHA would be given incentives for doing particular tasks. This reflected a broader trend of international initiatives (most of which focused on particular diseases) providing incentives for specific tasks related to their disease of interest—all while avoiding supporting the human resources of health systems in any broader way.[62]

So the ASHA was provided with incentives for carrying out particular activities, mostly related to maternal and child health. "They had a vision of her as a broker—a *tout*," one person familiar with the negotiations commented of those who created the ASHA program. But, they added, at least the incentives were "a way of getting past the government being unwilling to employ her."

Activism Despite the State

This incentive-based pay structure—which rewards ASHAs for specific tasks like childhood immunization and facility births, not broad based goals like community participation—reflects and reinforces the top down orientation of the ASHA program, as well as the metrics-focused orientation of global health broadly.[63] In other words, ASHAs are busy carrying out and quantifying specific tasks—like getting mothers to give birth in health facilities, getting babies into health centers for vaccination, and submitting reports showing the numbers of those tasks completed.

The tasks that an ASHA is reimbursed for, and the kinds of data she collates, are aimed at changing the behaviors of rural families in particular ways—for example, encouraging them to dramatically change rural Rajasthani family structure by having only two children.[64] These sets of tasks mirror those in CHW programs globally; many states want to change the behavior, particularly the reproductive behavior, of their rural populations through CHW programs.[65] They want to convince rural people to marry their daughters later, to use birth control, to educate their daughters, and to give birth in health facilities. These goals are shaped both by international metrics like the Sustainable Development Goals, and by government officials' own ideas of development and modernization.⁶⁶ India's policies for the ASHA program mirror these larger trends. As Sisdel Roalkvalm has observed, ASHAs are "both the objects and agents of development," expected to mold themselves and their neighbors in specific ways mandated by the state.⁶⁷

Although ASHA stands for "Accredited Social Health Activist," the "activist" part of the ASHA's work was not given the same attention as in the Mitanin program. While the Mitanin program had been run largely independently of state ministries, the ASHA would be part of the Ministry of Health, accountable to supervisors within that structure. Although there is a training module on activism in the official ASHA training materials, the ASHAs we knew had never seen it. In fact, they did not think that activism was part of their job responsibilities.

"The Indian state is extremely shrewd," someone who participated in the founding of the ASHA program commented. "They know how to say one thing and ensure that something else happens. They didn't want her to demand anything. The program is *designed* to keep her from being an activist. The state instituted education requirements: this is, of course, a proxy for class and caste."

In addition to the education requirements, ASHAs were required to be married—women in most parts of rural India move from the place they were born to live with their husband's family when they marry, and it may not always be appropriate for unmarried women to discuss topics like birth control. ASHAs' family involvement, too, could keep her from activism, the person who was active in the early program pointed out: "The daughter-in-law of a *sarpanch* (local elected official) is not likely to be an activist. She gets money for what the government wants her to do, not the village. Activism is a collective activity—so you would have to *support* community organizing for health."

Yet, both people we spoke to who were familiar with the founding of the program agreed, the creation of the ASHA program was a milestone. Although many ASHAs might be activists "despite the state," the program is nonetheless deeply meaningful: the largest system of CHWs in the world, around a million spanning the country.

And, the working conditions of ASHAs have had some political traction at the national level, with periodic discussions on how to better support ASHAs with pay and reasonable workloads.⁶⁸ Incentives have increased steadily over the years. So have ASHAs' responsibilities.

Beyond Lackeys and Liberators

This book builds on the existing literature on the political economy of health work through an exploration of two key aspects of CHW labor: first, the role that ASHAs' labor plays within their families; and second, the trajectory of their participation in unions. Both of these issues are central in understanding ASHAs' relationship to their work. Yet neither has thus far gotten much attention in either the anthropological or public health literature on CHWs.

We take as a starting point the important point, made in the anthropological literature on CHWs, that the lackey versus liberator dynamics are never quite so simple. CHWs are often both monitors of their neighbors' behavior and advocates for them.[69] And CHWs are diverse: their social, economic, and generational positions determine how they think about and enact their responsibilities, and CHW programs change over time.[70]

South Africa-based social scientists Chris Colvin and Alison Swartz have advised that anthropologists look beyond the top-down versus community-based models of CHW work, and instead understand CHWs "in community," through a model "that moves away from the individual and asks instead about the ways care work fits into broader social structures and processes more generally."[71] In this book, we aim to do just that for the ASHA program. In doing so, we build on existing literature, including the work of anthropologists like Kenneth Maes who have so clearly outlined the ways that volunteer CHW labor can be exploitative.[72] In this book, we explore additional social dimensions of CHW work: ASHAs' relationships within families and within labor unions. These social dimensions are deeply gendered. They also illuminate the multifaceted nature of CHW work for ASHAs, and show how the work transforms their lives in complex ways.

The literature on ASHAs is voluminous: a recent review identified 122 articles written on the program.[73] Within this literature, several excellent pieces situate the ASHAs' work in Rajasthan within social relations in the health system, and within community hierarchies.[74] As Nordfeldt and Roalkvam show, the government's promotional material notwithstanding, the ASHA is not a "health sister," she is rather "a *village* sister, participating in the local social games of relations and hierarchy."[75]

For ASHAs in Rajasthan, one critical village relationship was the one they had with Anganwadi Workers, village-level female volunteer workers focused on child nutrition. The relationships between ASHAs and Anganwadi Workers—and other co-workers and supervisors—are sometimes fraught, and tied to their families' statuses in the community.[76] As in the vignette above where Meena argued with her supervisors, relationships between different cadres of workers can be hierarchical and sometimes strained.

These hierarchies are not just in health systems: they are also in families, where the young women who are often chosen as CHWs are typically low-status members. Yet across the literature on ASHAs and Anganwadi Workers—and indeed the literature on CHWs around the world—the role of CHWs' families remains largely unexplored. Many researchers, particularly in India, are well aware that families are important: Kavita Bhatia, for example, describes ASHAs' families in Maharashtra as "an uncounted stakeholder."[77] By this Bhatia means that ASHAs' families shape their work and the program in significant ways. However, these dynamics remain for the most part mentioned only in passing.

In part this may be because of an unhelpful conceptual distinction between "work" and what many people in the United States often call "life" (meaning everything outside of work). But for the ASHAs we knew, this distinction was not neat at all. At home, the labor burden of many of the ASHAs we knew was crushing. As we describe in this book, going to work as an ASHA was for some women a break from the work at home. And the very fact that they were ASHAs at all was almost always because of family ties and family decisions. The stories in this book show that for ASHAs, CHW work could not be separated out from family relations.

This book also explores the social entanglements of ASHAs in union structures. Although CHWs across the world are involved in unions, our understanding of what really happens within unions, the social and power relations involved, and the implications for health systems is still nascent.[78] Some recently published work has suggested that the impact of CHW unionization may be limited in many contexts.[79] In South Africa, the fragility of emerging CHW unions, as well as opposition from the South African Ministry of Health, has thus far kept CHW organizing from making significant headway.[80] Our goal was to understand these dynamics in India, to flesh out CHW work and the complexity of its power relations and politics.[81]

We went into this research with a range of questions about the social context of community health work: How does this work shift gender relations within the family? How and when do ASHAs push back against power structures in the family, and in the health system, and what happens when they do? Are unions a way of shifting these power dynamics, and what might the complicated unintended consequences of unionization be?

In this book, we tell the story of ASHAs' families, and ASHAs' unions, from the ASHAs' point of view. Our telling of these stories would be different if we had spent most of our time with supervisors, policymakers, or union leaders. We interviewed all of those people, but we did not spend our days with them. The focus of this book is on ASHAs' central concerns. So, for example, this book is not really about whether ASHAs are doing a good job at their work (a concern of many supervisors and policymakers). Instead, this book is about what the ASHAs we came to know and admire wanted us to write about.

These stories are complex. Working as an ASHA changed these women's lives and relationships in profound ways; but there are no easy narratives of "empowerment" here. Nor do narratives of neoliberalism or biopower—two anthropological frames often applied in analyses of global health programs—paint the full picture.[82] The structure of ASHA work was shaped in part by neoliberal forces—as can be seen in the reluctance to provide ASHAs with a salaried position, and in the incentive-based pay structure that was implemented instead. And biopower—the diffuse and complex ways that people's very bodies are shaped by powerful global forces—is at work in the program. This can be seen in what those incentives reward: encouraging smaller families, and promoting specific practices of immunization and child feeding. Yet these forces explain only a piece of what is going on for the ASHAs we know.

In this book, we go deeper into how ASHA work changed the trajectory of young women's lives in rural Rajasthan in meaningful and complicated ways. These changes were something much more complex and more interesting than either exploitation or empowerment. Despite the undoubtedly top-down nature of the program, ASHAs were not just cogs in the machine (although they complained that they felt that way sometimes). In addition, the work was profoundly transformative in various ways for ASHAs themselves.

Early chapters of this book explore how ASHA work intersected with young women's positions as young daughters-in-law, and how working as an ASHA changed their relationships with their families, and also their views of the world.

In the later chapters of the book, we describe what happened when, after experiencing these transformations, women began to advocate for themselves, within the health system, and through unions. There, they encountered power structures that were very slow to bend.

The ASHAs who are featured in this book opened up their lives to us, and were generous with their time and their energy, because they had something important to say, and they saw us as a conduit to saying it. They were not shy about telling us *that* was the deal: they would help us tell the stories of their lives in all their messiness and complexity; we would write a book that would show the world that they deserved more respect, and more power. Our job—a job that is taking us far too long according to the ASHAs involved—is to tell their stories in a way that does them some justice. We hope that we have communicated the passion, commitment, humor, and luminous intelligence of these women, and that we have passed on a bit of the enormous respect we have for them.

Methods: Following the Threads of ASHA Activism

There were ten ASHAs in Gurha Sajjanpura. There were also ten Anganwadi Workers and "Anganwadi Helpers," other women who work on child nutrition. The Anganwadi Workers and Anganwadi Helpers were employed at Anganwadi Centers, child care centers that provided preschool education and nutrition supplements. All of these groups of women were "voluntary" workers, none provided with minimum wage or job security. The Anganwadi Workers were all educated; they taught the preschool classes and made a bit more than ASHAs.

The Anganwadi Helper position did not require literacy; these women cooked food for the children and helped clean the center. Anganwadi Helpers earned least of all, and many of these women were living in total poverty. They had often been given the Anganwadi Helper position by community leaders as a way of providing some limited income support after they had been widowed or abandoned by their husbands' families.

In 2018 and 2019, we interviewed all thirty of these women. We also interviewed the families of five of these ASHAs, five Anganwadi Workers, and three Anganwadi Helpers. These family interviews varied in format. Some were one-on-one interviews with the worker's husband or father-in-law, but in most cases when we visited workers' homes, we found that many family members were curious about our project and interested in providing their perspectives; they often wanted to discuss our questions with us as a group. In cases where they preferred it, we conducted group interviews with families—discussions that lasted one to two hours and often included both male and female family members spanning two generations. All participants provided informed consent, and we audio recorded the interviews.

We also conducted participant observation in many settings around Gurha Sajjanpura. We stayed in town, with local families, while we conducted our fieldwork. We attended ASHA trainings and meetings. We spent time at the health center during immunization days and accompanied ASHAs on their home visits with families. We spent mornings at the Anganwadi Centers. And we participated in local events, from festivals to children's birthday parties. We took detailed fieldnotes during participant observation.

Our work was based in the community, but overall, it focused on ASHAs. It was ASHAs' concerns and workloads and experiences that were the heart of the work, not the experiences of the community members they served. Those voices are also important, of course. But every research project has to make choices about where to bound the work, and we focused on ASHA experiences because we felt that doing so provided a particularly fascinating and revealing entry point for institutional ethnography—understanding the complex workings of the state and international agencies from the vantage point of ASHAs was our overall goal. This provides a complement, not a replacement, to the huge body of anthropological work focused on the experiences of clients of health systems.[83] In this book, we center the experiences of the ASHA.

While our work started in Gurha Sajjanpura, it did not end there. Following the threads of ASHAs' activism took us to the city of Jaipur. Tourists from around the world flock to Jaipur for its spectacular ancient forts and palaces. But most of the ASHAs we worked with had never been to these sites—they visited Jaipur to attend trainings, or to attend union rallies and sit-ins. We joined the ASHAs at these union activities in Jaipur, talking to ASHAs, to police, and to union leaders, and sitting with them as they protested. We took fieldnotes during this participant observation.

At these events in Jaipur, we met influential ASHAs we had heard talked about in Gurha Sajjanpura, women who had organized other ASHAs and who were seen as leaders. Meena was one of those women. With their collaboration, we followed those women, too, learning more about their lives and visiting the towns where they lived and worked. We conducted in-depth interviews with these women, often multiple times. We also interviewed key union leaders.

This project was supposed to wrap up in summer 2020—but the COVID pandemic altered both our plans and those of the ASHAs we knew. This project sat on hold for a few years. In 2022 and 2023, after the pandemic's restrictions on our work were eased, we conducted follow-up interviews with ten of these ASHAs. It has been a true joy to connect with them repeatedly and follow them over five years.

"Something Could Change"

"My family says this: the biggest thing I've gotten from my job is an expanded awareness," Meena explained. Navigating travel outside of town—to obtain goods or heath care—was something that was usually reserved for men in Rajasthani families. But thanks to her ASHA work, Meena had become so much more comfortable with the broader world than the men in her family that she was doing it now.

"Actually, I understand so much that I have taken over a lot of the family travel from my husband," Meena told us. "If we need to visit somewhere, or get something, I will go—spend the night, come back the next day. My husband tells me to get a motor scooter—I say, I don't make that much!"

She laughed, but turned serious when considering the road ahead, toward unionizing, advocating for a living wage, a real job. "All of the ASHAs will have to work together. Otherwise, it doesn't matter what you do, nothing will happen. If all the ASHAs work together, something could change. I am ready."

CHAPTER 2

We Talk to Everyone

The Work of an ASHA

Bharti, an ASHA in Gurha Sajjanpura, had always been an avid gardener, but during COVID she really leaned into it. Her modest three-room house opened onto an outdoor courtyard, packed with thriving potted plants large and small. Some were useful as herbal remedies; some were beautiful; some, Bharti explained with her big smile, just looked interesting. Before COVID, we used to sit on her bed in one of her small rooms and chat with her. After COVID, we would sit among the plants outside and drink tea while we talked.

Bharti was the only ASHA in Gurha Sajjanpura who didn't live with her extended family. In an unusual move, she and her husband had left the house they had shared with his parents, and struck out on their own. That had been years ago—they had left when Bharti's first daughter was a toddler, and her second daughter hadn't even been born yet. Now both her daughters had master's degrees. Bharti, herself only educated to the twelfth grade, had come a long way.

It had been a long, hard road though. Money had always been scarce. Bharti's husband worked as a salesperson in a grocery stall, making Rs 8,000 (about $100) a month. Since they had left the extended family, they didn't have any land, so no food or income could come from farming.

"I'm telling you, I work so hard!" Bharti said, laughing. When she and her husband had first moved to Gurja Sajjanpura, she made jewelry from home in an attempt to make extra money. Then, she learned to sew, got a sewing machine, and began tailoring clothes for local women. And she took up ASHA work when it became available. It was all part of her ongoing hustle to create a pleasant home and to educate her daughters.

"We all used to work together," Bharti said, thinking back to the years when her daughters were younger. "Their father would go to earn money, and the girls would go to school, but the girls also worked hard in the morning and the evening." Bharti herself worked hardest of all: getting up early in the morning to make the day's food, do the housework, and care for the cow before she had to head off for her ASHA work.

The ASHA work itself, Bharti commented, didn't make a lot of sense in terms of her overall income. Laughing, she commented that one of her friends had asked her, "Why are you doing this job? You're not getting anything! You make better money at home."

But it wasn't just about the money. Yes, she was hopeful that someday the pay would increase. But Bharti's motivation was deeper, she explained to us:

> I built this house. I don't have enough money for the roof—so I just used corrugated metal! I don't really have much furniture either—I just cover my clothes with a sheet! I have three rooms and one kitchen, but no stairs. My house isn't yet complete. But, my daughters have studied well.
>
> Some women, they are just living, and they don't know anything about the outside world. If I didn't do this job, I'd also be like them. They haven't had a chance to consider what they want out of life. And what could be more important than that? There's so much more out there than doing housework and making dinner.

"Those Days, They Won't Come Again"

To understand the social context of ASHA work, it's helpful to look at the defined life trajectory for Hindu women in rural Rajasthan. The life trajectories of Gurha Sajjanpura's ASHAs unfolded in a series of very distinct stages.

All of the ASHAs in Gurha Sajjanpura were Hindu (despite the fact that there was a sizable Muslim minority in town). Since the ASHA position had educational requirements, the ASHAs all also came from families with enough money to educate them, meaning they were not from the poorest families. At each stage of their lives, these women had different responsibilities, opportunities, and freedoms.

From birth until their marriage, women lived primarily with their parents, almost always in their fathers' extended families—with grandparents, aunts and uncles, and many cousins sharing a home or a group of homes. In the village or town they were born in, they were a "sister of the whole village"—they moved freely, and the ideology, at least, was that everyone would look out for them.

Most girls and unmarried women in Gurha Sajjanpura wear the same clothes as their age-mates in the cities: cute dresses when they are young, and as they get older, stylish jeans and tops. They do not veil, and they speak freely at home. They have relatively few responsibilities: they may help out with cooking or fieldwork, to a greater or lesser degree depending on the family's needs, but they are not seen as primarily responsible for these tasks. These young women have many freedoms—for example, they can travel freely with other young women, even taking the bus to nearby cities. If the family can afford it, women at this stage in their lives might be sent to a city for their higher education, where they might live with relatives or in a university hostel.

Marriage brought on a dramatic change in the lives of Gurha Sajjanpura's ASHAs and Anganwadi Workers. Being married was a requirement for getting one of these jobs—both to ensure that they would stay in town long-term, and that they would have the necessary status to talk to married women about issues of family planning and childbirth.

When they were married, all of the women we interviewed moved out of their parents' village and into a new village or town to live with their new husband's family. In some cases, the young woman knew her husband and may have pushed for the match—in other cases, her parents chose him, and she did not know him at all before moving into his home. But in any case, ASHAs' husbands were not the only, or often even the primary, social relationship in their new homes: the contours of their new life were often largely set by their mothers- and fathers-in-law.

In a young Hindu Rajasthani bride's new home, a comprehensive set of rules about veiling, modesty, and seclusion—*ghūṅghaṭa*—apply. Women leave jeans and t-shirts for saris or *ghagra cholis*—beautiful clothes with yards of fabric that signal her adult status. Young married women commonly veil completely in front of their male relatives in their husband's house and in their husband's town, pulling their saris or scarves down to completely cover their faces. (These rules are quite different from veiling traditions in Muslim communities in South Asia, where women do not veil inside the house with their families or their husband's families.) Young married Hindu women in Rajasthan also speak in a whisper in front of male relatives and their mothers-in-law; sit physically below male relatives and their mothers-in-law, choosing the ground if those people are on chairs; and limit their mobility outside the home to essential tasks only. The embodiment of these rules is comprehensive: young married women in Gurja Sajjanpura constantly adjust themselves in space depending on who can see them. We watched ASHAs' body language change completely when a male relative entered the room, and when ASHAs passed men on village paths.

The extent to which these guidelines actually apply varies from house to house, and women stretch these boundaries in all kinds of ways.[1] As we will explore in the next chapters, ASHA work changed these rules significantly. Still, many ASHAs who were animated and voluble at the Anganwadi Centers remained completely silent when we visited them at home.

Young married women in Gurha Sajjanpura go back and visit their parents frequently, particularly when they are having their first child. In their natal homes, they regain some of their old freedoms. But the shift is nonetheless profound. "Those days, they won't come again," one young married woman in Gurha Sajjanpura mused wistfully about her time in college, when she had lived in a hostel with her classmates in a major city.

In their new families, young married women are generally low-status members expected to do a great deal of work. Under the supervision of their mother-in-law, these women typically manage a heavy work burden.

We asked all of our interviewees about the structure of their days. ASHAs' responses were quite consistent. Nearly all of Gurha Sajjanpura's ASHAs got up around 4 a.m. Most began their day by collecting manure from the cattle; making tea and food for the entire household; and packing lunches for the children that were going to school. They cleaned the house, woke their children, and prepared them for school. Then, they left the house in order to get to work at the Anganwadi Center.

When their ASHA work was done (usually around noon or one, but occasionally substantially later), these women went home and ate lunch. They fed their preschool children and stole their few moments of rest in the day, napping or scrolling on a phone if they had one. Then, they washed the lunch dishes by hand, washed the clothes for everyone in the household by hand, worked in the fields for several hours, tended and milked the animals, cooked dinner for everyone, worked with the school-aged children on their homework, cleaned up the dinner dishes, and hoped to make it into bed by 10 p.m.

This relentless work structure would last for years. But it would not shape the rest of their lives.

As a woman ages and younger women marry into the household, her status increases. The most dramatic status change for married women in Gurha Sajjanpura occurs when their *sons* get married. Some older Anganwadi Workers had married sons; their workloads were much more relaxed. With daughters-in-law of their own to do the work of the household, these women's roles shifted from labor to supervision. Rather than cooking food, washing dishes and clothes, and working in the fields, these older women advised and supervised their daughters-in-law in carrying out these tasks. An older woman's workload decreases; her power increases.

Along with these changes in power come changes in veiling and mobility. Middle-aged women in Gurha Sajjanpura still veil symbolically in front of older family members, but the rules surrounding veiling and mobility relax progressively as women age and gain status. Women in their forties commonly speak in confident voices in all settings. And although they are still less mobile than men, they move quite freely around town without asking for permission.

Throughout all of these changes, there was a powerful throughline—*izzat*, or honor. Married women were expected to behave in ways that upheld the honor of their families. Maintaining honor—both for the family and the woman herself—held deep and profound social importance.

"Why Are You Repeatedly Coming to Our Door?"

Once COVID hit, things were very tough for Bharti. Gurha Sajjanpura, like the rest of Rajasthan, had extremely strict lockdown measures in the early days of the pandemic. There was one worker, however, who was expected to go door to door, delivering supplies and checking for COVID cases: the ASHA.

ASHAs across India went door to door to every house in the country. They found out who had symptoms, and who had come to the village from outside. They didn't have tests; those were available at the quarantine center that had been set up at the local school. All they could do was tell people about COVID and tell them to isolate. Bharti told us about it.

> It was difficult. The hospital was telling us to go out and do community surveys. Go and tell everyone not to leave their houses. Tell everyone to wash their hands, maintain social distancing, keep themselves away from the cold. We told everyone these things, going door to door. But some people said, "Madam, we know these things. Why are you repeatedly coming to our door? You are going to give us Corona."

Some people also said, "Do you actually have any test kits? If so, please tell us. And test us now for Corona." And I would say, "I have nothing. I have to send you to the hospital for that."

If I was thirsty, nobody would offer me water. In those Corona times, nobody offered. Nobody wanted to touch me, nobody wanted me to get close. Nobody offered me a chair, and nobody was ready to talk. If I was speaking, someone would answer me from far away. "Why did you come here?"

We did this for a long time. Until there was a vaccine, and until the vaccine was delivered, we continuously did surveys.

When the ASHAs found a probable COVID case, they would tell their supervisors. Then, the person would be called to the school for testing. If the test came back positive, the ASHA would be sent to bring that person to quarantine. This was a very difficult job for the ASHA, who did not have a lot of power to tell older people or men in her village what to do. But, they were the ones in the field. "In that time, the only ones who went out door to door, in the village, it was us, right?" Bharti commented. "So the reporting for the entire village, it all came from us ASHAs."

In Gurha Sajjanpura, quarantine was initially at the school, but over time home quarantine was increasingly allowed, using the school facility only if there wasn't space in someone's home for them to quarantine. Every day, one ASHA explained, they would check back in with the family, and "check in with the patient, are they still testing positive, do they have any problems, do they need to be referred to the hospital." Bharti explained that she would give the COVID-positive person a care kit from the hospital. And at the end of the quarantine period, she would let them know that they could leave.

ASHAs also had to tell anyone who had come into Gurha Sajjanpura from outside to quarantine, either at home or at the school. This was really difficult for Bharti. Her supervisors at the hospital were insistent that she find visitors and tell them to quarantine. Since the quarantine center obviously was a high risk place for COVID, most people didn't want to go. So the people Bharti was directing to quarantine were often angry. And Bharti herself was stuck in the middle.

"People were really afraid," Bharti explained. "And they would get upset: 'Why are you stopping us here [at the quarantine center]? We came from so far away only to see our family members—and you are keeping us from doing that! What do you hospital people want?'" There was no way to fix this situation.

Every ASHA we asked about their time during COVID talked about fear: how scared they were going door to door, how scared their families were. They all laughed when recalling these things, but it wasn't really funny. It was more of: what can you do?

"I don't know what kind of debts I incurred in the last life," one ASHA commented, laughing, "that I have this much opportunity to do service in this one."

"Yes, I was afraid," Bharti told us. "But what to do? It was my duty. I had to go. And my supervisors had put so much pressure on me!"

She added, laughing, "sometimes my husband, he would say, 'What kind of job is this? Put yourself in danger, put your children in danger, get everyone in the house sick, and go around helping other people.'"

Bharti was, again, caught in the middle.

"Grab Them However You Can"

When the vaccine became available, again the ASHAs had a central role. They were among the first to be vaccinated, given priority as medical professionals. To some ASHAs, this felt like much needed recognition. But this was mixed with anxiety. Another ASHA named Kavita commented, again laughing: "I got the vaccine, first. The first of anyone. They gave it to ASHAs first. Because, we were going to the field. Yes, by all means, give it to us! If we die, then you all will know it's not safe!"

When more vaccine became available, ASHAs were responsible for organizing people to be vaccinated: to identify who was eligible, to let those people know where to go. At first, ASHAs had to navigate scarcity; there was not enough vaccine for everyone. They had to let people know who was eligible, setting people's expectations and helping the elderly navigate long lines. Over time, they had to navigate opposition, trying to convince people to be vaccinated.

Every ASHA talked about the intense pressure they faced during this time from their supervisors at the health post. One explained:

> They told us: "The vaccine has come. You have to bring fifty people, by any means." By any means at all! We were so pressured. "Grab them however you can. We shouldn't send any vaccine back." They put an unbelievable amount of pressure on us. To use every last bit of vaccine. If there were any doses left in the vial, find ten more people.
>
> They made us work by threatening us.

While the ASHAs were pressured by their supervisors to deliver people to get vaccinated, they also faced resistance from some people who were frightened that the vaccine would harm them. ASHAs often used their own example in these cases: "I'm not dead! I got the vaccine and I'm still here!" Kavita said she would tell people. Sometimes they soft-pedaled the side effects. Bharti commented, "I didn't tell anyone I got a fever from the vaccine! I didn't want people in the village to be afraid."

But finally, the ASHAs told us, almost everyone in Gurha Sajjanpura was vaccinated, something they were proud of. "In the end," Bharti said, "everyone was ready to vaccinate."

The ASHAs we spoke to were justly proud of the work they did during COVID. One commented:

> The government benefited so much from us. Otherwise, the ANMs and the doctors were definitely not going to go door to door! They would never go. The doctors, if you called them to see a COVID patient, they might come but they would just look at the patient from far away. But the ASHAs don't think like that. We don't talk from far away. We always go in the house and talk to everyone.
>
> Without the ASHAs, there wouldn't have been that much vaccination for Corona. It wasn't happening. It was because of the hard work of ASHAs that people were getting vaccinated. If they refused, we would explain to them.

"I was afraid," Bharti said, "but the work had to get done. Otherwise, Corona was going to spread. How would the village be spared from Corona?"

Everyone worked hard, she explained, "but the main work was for the ASHA." And, she noted, although the door to door work was the most emotionally weighty, the paperwork was perhaps the most onerous part of the job during COVID. "We had to fill out so many forms!" There were forms for COVID patients, forms for tracking who had come from outside the village.

But this was nothing new. Filling out forms had always been a central part of the ASHA job.

"I Helped Her with the Paperwork"

On a sunny July morning back in 2019, Kavita headed out for her door-to-door ASHA visits (fig. 2.1). We were going with her. "You'll understand my work better if you walk with me," Kavita had told us, adding the caution, "It's far!"

Kavita was young, in her early twenties. When she started work as an

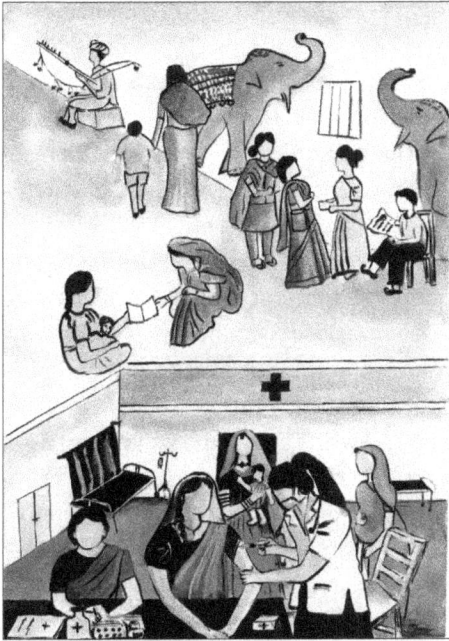

FIGURE 2.1. Kavita at work. At the top, she travels around the village counseling women and helping with their paperwork. In the lower scene, she keeps records at the health post while the ANM gives vaccinations. Illustration © Soniya Kanwar.

ASHA, she was only tenth-grade educated, but now she had a master's degree that she had gotten from correspondence courses. Kavita was from a relatively wealthy family in Gurha Sajjanpura; she always dressed beautifully, today in a vivid green sari edged with a silver ribbon.

In July in Gurha Sajjanpura, the brutal heat of May and June begins to break, with the arrival of the torrential afternoon downpours of the monsoon. We followed Kavita along a dirt road, a fence of thorns protecting a field on one side. The sun was punishing, but Kavita commented that the walk was not so bad now that the monsoon had started. "Once on this road, the heat was so bad, and I had no water, and I started to cry!"

After walking a kilometer or so, we reached a house, set back from the road amid bright green fields. As we turned toward it, Kavita pulled the end of her beautiful sari down over her face, obscuring herself completely.

The grandmother of the household, who was sitting in the outdoor courtyard, greeted Kavita warmly, welcomed us, and called out to the two young women of the household, her grandsons' wives. The young women came out, saris also pulled down over their faces, greeting Kavita quietly and politely. One of them was pregnant; the other held a small girl.

"I helped her with the paperwork," Kavita explained. "To get her pay- ments." Because this woman had a girl child, she was eligible for finan- cial incentives from the government. For immunizing and educating her daughter, she received substantial payments—payments not available to parents of boys.

"Girls can be a burden," the grandmother explained to us. "This makes them less of a burden." A major goal of the *Mukhyamantree Rājśrī Yojanā* program is to close the mortality gap between girls and boys in Rajasthan, which is wide. Boys have better survival rates than girls, largely because daughters, with their huge dowry requirements, are truly enormous finan- cial burdens on families—while sons, who will *receive* dowries when they get married, and will stay with the family they are born into, generally improve a family's economic situation long-term. In situations of extreme poverty, having mostly daughters can be disastrous for the well-being of the family as a whole. And, through a steady accumulation of subtle ways that families prefer boys, these dynamics add up to worse health outcomes for girl chil- dren. The financial incentives from the government are designed to make raising a daughter less financially painful for impoverished families—and, hopefully, to improve female survival and education rates.

These financial incentives are meaningful for families. But obtaining them, Kavita explained to us, was complex, with many bureaucratic steps that could be difficult for illiterate women. First, the mother needed to have an *aadhaar* card—a national ID card. Often, these cards still had the address of the woman's parents, and needed to be changed to reflect the address of her marital family. The ASHA helped women with that.

Next, women needed a ration card, a way of getting government food aid. The ASHA helped with that, too.

Women also needed a *bhamashah* card, a type of family health incentive card issued by the Government of Rajasthan only to women, with payments going to the woman's account. Some women still did not have *bhamashah* cards when they first became pregnant. And yes, Kavita added, she helped women get their *bhamashah* cards.

In order to get the *bhamashah* card, though, the women first needed a bank account. Most women did not have accounts in their own names. So ASHAs helped with that, too.

The ASHA also filled out a *mamta* card for pregnant women; it was a booklet that tracked their prenatal checkups, as well as their child's health care and growth.

Once women had all of those items, they could begin to get some of their incentives. Even then, to actually get the incentives, they needed to submit yet more paperwork—for example, paperwork showing that their daughters had been immunized. The ASHAs filled out all the forms, Kavita explained, and *then* the money went into the mother's account.

As we sipped tea at the house, there was discussion of one child's ringworm infection. They had sought treatment at the health center, and the medicine had worked for a while, but now the itching was back. The grandmother asked Kavita what to do; Kavita didn't know, and didn't pretend to. She advised the family to go back to the health center.

Then the conversation turned back to paperwork. Kavita explained in detail to the young mother about the documents she needed to file, including some steps that had to be done online. Kavita outlined all of the steps for the forms that needed to be filled out, the photocopies that needed to be made. If Kavita was not an authority on ringworm, she was an absolute authority when it came to bureaucracy.

"Everyone Treats Me Well Here"

We went on to the next house—this one had a painted cement gate, and two *charpoys* (rope and wood beds) in the courtyard. A young woman greeted us familiarly—she also knew Kavita—and invited us into the main room, a large, spare space with brick walls. Birds chirped from the rafters. There were two babies at this house, both enormous cute chubby round six-month-olds. They knew Kavita and laughed when she scooped them up; they eyed both of us warily, though.

The babies' mothers brought out some documents for Kavita to look over. As she did so, Kavita told them it was time to start giving the babies some solid food and told them when the babies should get immunized next. As she worked, one of the babies' mothers made us tea, her sari obscuring her face.

"Everyone treats me well here," Kavita commented. "They understand that I'm doing my job, that I'm helping them." Before she started working as an ASHA, Kavita knew this family a little. At that time, though, she "never left the house" because of restrictions on her movement, so she had no chance to get to know them well. Now that she visited for ASHA work, the friendship had grown. The friendship had genuine warmth; it was good to see the two of them together.

Surendra and the men of the house moved into the other room, and Kavita, the two young mothers, and Svea moved into the kitchen, now an all-female space. The young women immediately took their saris off of their heads, and the quiet figures transformed into gregarious personalities. They brought the conversation around to family planning—a topic never discussed when men were in the room—explaining confidently and comfortably, and with a bit of humor, what local women saw as the pros and cons of the various methods the ASHA offered. These women preferred condoms, and Kavita provided them.

Svea asked Kavita if she needed to weigh the babies—growth charts being a big part of the data Kavita needed to submit. "Look at these babies!" Kavita cried, gesturing toward the plump, healthy kids—who, it was true, were definitely not underweight. "In our area there aren't any underweight ones! Yes, if they're premature, then you should measure them." Kavita took a pragmatic approach to the work she was asked to do, skipping some tasks (weighing babies) if she saw them as unnecessary, and spending an enormous amount of time on tasks that were not part of her official job description (compiling and filing paperwork to get women official identity cards and bank accounts).

Kavita was typical in allocating her time this way. The bulk of ASHAs' work in Gurha Sajjanpura—and the task that was seen as most helpful by the women they served—was assisting women in navigating bureaucracies, from filling out the paperwork needed to access government benefits, to helping them make their way through confusing urban hospitals. In part, this was because for the women ASHAs served, filing paperwork was necessary to get cash incentives from the government for activities like vaccinating baby girls. It was also critical for the ASHAs themselves—if their clients' paperwork was not correct, the ASHAs would not get incentive payments for the services they assisted with. Sometimes ASHAs performed this work themselves; in other cases, they advised families on how to do those tasks. The people that ASHAs served were grateful for this work.

"People Get Frustrated with the Bureaucracy"

The health center in Gurha Sajjanpura was a pleasant place: light, with tiled floors and walls. We arrived at 9 a.m. one Thursday morning in 2019, a little before the center really got busy. The Auxiliary Nurse-Midwife (ANM), who lived in a nearby city, was already there, getting set up in the hallway and entering information into a huge register. The ANM, unlike the ASHAs, had a permanent government position, with higher pay, job security, and benefits. She was above the ASHAs in the very hierarchical hospital system.

Near the ANM, a woman sat on a bench and sorted through a huge stack of papers; she was getting ready to file the necessary *Mukhyamantree Rājśrī Yojanā* paperwork for her daughter. Her son, a cute grinning boy of four or five, eagerly helped her organize the papers. At long last, she got her paperwork in order and gave it to the ANM. The ANM glanced at it, handed it back to her, and told her to wait—she was busy filling out the register.

When it was her turn, the ANM looked over all of the paperwork, organized it, got her to sign it, told her to get a photocopy of the documents from the market, and then to submit all of the documents to the computer operator—who had his own room across the hall, with the health post's only computer in it.

"I've been to so many shops, the electricity is out at all of them," the woman complained, but headed out anyway to attempt to find a working photocopier somewhere in town.

When she returned, the ANM and the computer operator examined and discussed her bank paperwork. The computer operator collated the documents that were needed for her to get her benefits: an *aadhaar* card; a bank passbook; a discharge ticket from her hospital birth; and a photocopy of her *mamta* card.

"People get frustrated with the bureaucracy," the ANM commented to us, "but the ASHA and I, we both follow up with them. I call them on the phone, the ASHA visits them in person."

This Thursday was an immunization day in Gurha Sajjanpura, an event that happened once a month. The hallway was starting to fill up, a line forming in front of the ANM, who had set up a table with vaccines in coolers and a stack of disposable syringes. A gap-toothed toddler, who was accompanied by her very pregnant mother, proudly showed us the two rupees her parents had given her as an enticement to be vaccinated. When it was the toddler's turn, the ANM took the vaccines from the cooler on the table—a specially designed one with depressions in it to hold the vials—and with swift, practiced movements, opened a disposable syringe, filled it with vaccine, and vaccinated the toddler. The girl screamed loudly with her first shot, and even louder with her second, while the ANM handed a few pain relief tablets to her mother, instructing her to give them to the child if, and only if, she had pain and fever.

While the ANM was vaccinating children, a skeletally thin man entered and stood in the hallway, wearing a face mask. Seeing him, the ANM got out special vials with powder in them, carefully adding water to reconstitute his medicine. The ANM explained that this man had multi-drug resistant tuberculosis (MDRTB)—to treat his strain of the disease meant providing expensive drugs that previously had been all but unavailable. But now there was a program to get the extraordinarily expensive, lifesaving drugs to MDRTB patients free of cost through the health center. Although the ANM was helping monitor the medication at the health post, ASHAs also followed up with these patients.

The man was a cement laborer, and we knew that one of his co-workers had recently died—likely also of MDTRB. Without the medication that the ANM was preparing, this man would probably die too.

Immunization Data

Around 10 a.m., Kavita arrived, along with two other ASHAs. The ANM scolded them as they came through the door: "You're so late! I was so stressed—here all by myself."

The ASHAs laughed, each blaming her lateness on the other. The ANM, scolding them again sternly, moved on to explaining to the ASHAs how to fill out the huge registers spread out on a table next to her. As parents came through the line, the ASHAs recorded the weights of pregnant women and toddlers using a scale.

Three more ASHAs showed up, including Bharti; half of Gurha Sajjanpura's ASHAs were now present to help. (The other five would come for the next immunization day.) The paperwork required all five ASHAs' full attention. Two ASHAs checked everyone in on one side of the line; the ANM gave the vaccinations and entered some information into a register of her own; and then the other ASHAs copied information from the *mamta* card into three places: two health center registers, and the ASHAs' own booklets where they tracked all the parents in their catchment area. Kavita did this in a notebook, explaining, "This is just rough work—I'll copy it nicely into the final register later."

One woman had showed up with a newborn but without a *bhamashah* card; the ANM carefully coached her and her husband on how to obtain one, and in the meantime the ASHAs worked out how to enter her materials properly into the various registers.

Some cases were complex. For example, a grandmother came in with her infant granddaughter, asking how to get her registered for the *Mukhyamantree Rājśrī Yojanā* payments. There was a problem with the payments, because the father of the baby had kicked the mother out of the house. The mother had taken the baby with her, but the official paperwork still listed the baby as living with her father (the usual pattern in Rajasthan). This made paperwork a challenge: the ASHAs patiently walked her through the steps she would need to take to submit the necessary paperwork in the child's father's village.

For many other complex paperwork issues, the ANMs and ASHAs, busy as they were at the moment, told parents to follow up with the ASHAs later, when they would have more time to help.

Eventually the line began to wind down. The group had seen more than thirty-five families that morning, and by 12:30, it was quiet. The ANM and two ASHAs were left with paperwork in the main room, and the other three ASHAs congregated in the computer room to submit their information into the lone computer. The Internet wasn't working at the moment, so their supervisor was entering everything into Excel; she would have to copy it onto a web form later. By one o'clock, the ASHAs began to head back home.

"We Have 100 Children"

Before the pandemic, the ASHAs not only worked on collating health data, they also worked on collating data on nutrition for the local Anganwadi Center, a place that provided child care and nutrition services to children in the community. Every Anganwadi Center had female community workers as well—they taught preschool concepts to children and provided them with food.

At every Anganwadi Center, there were around twenty separate registers that had to be maintained by the ASHAs and the Anganwadi Workers (fig. 2.2).

Bharti sat with us one day in 2018 at her Anganwadi Center, fanned out the registers in front of us, and went over them. The data that ASHAs and

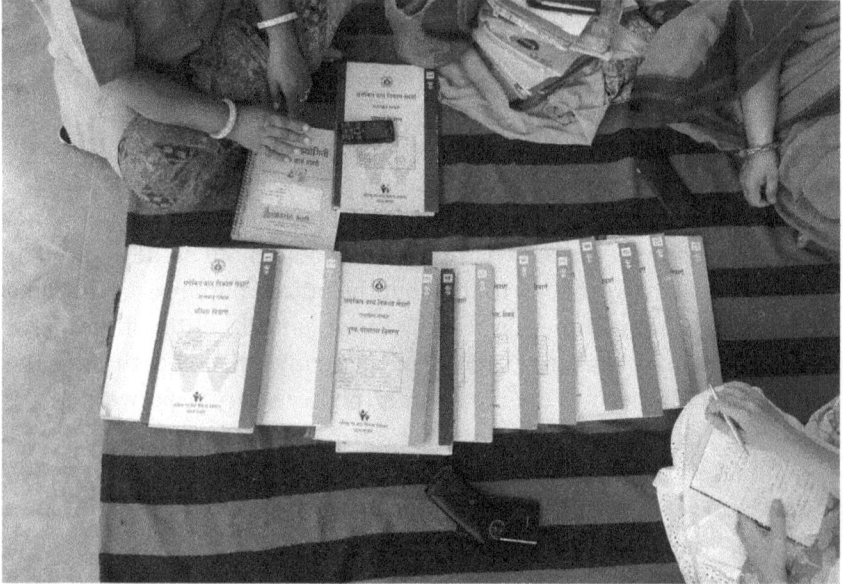

FIGURE 2.2. Bharti's data registers. She exclaimed, "There are boxes of registers! There are more inside." Photo by Surendra Shekhawat.

Anganwadi Workers were expected to keep current in separate registers included:

- The ASHA diary, a complete compilation of all of the ASHAs' tasks
- A complete list of everyone in the catchment area of the Anganwadi Center, including a comprehensive list of births and deaths: Kavita's center served 152 houses, with 223 families—a total population of around 1,200 people
- Another register summarizing this information by household
- A separate summary birth register
- Growth charts for every child in the area
- A separate register with the weights of every child
- A register of pregnant women, including information on maternal immunization and interventions like iron supplementation
- A record of Vitamin A supplementation for all the children in the area
- A daily log of which children came to the Anganwadi Center for preschool

- A register of the food given to the children at the Anganwadi Center, with daily details
- A summary register of the food given
- A referral log for children who need health interventions
- A home visit register for pregnant women, documenting the ASHAs' prenatal care visits (seven visits for each pregnant woman)
- A register of supervisory visits by the Anganwadi Supervisor
- A register for the *sarpanch*, a local political leader, including mobile phone numbers of everyone in the area, and information on whether each family had received certain government benefits

"Look at all this work, and how low our salary is!" the Anganwadi Worker who worked with Bharti exclaimed. "We have one hundred children!"

The amount of paperwork that ASHAs and Anganwadi Workers were managing—some of which was officially their responsibility, and some that was officially the responsibility of their supervisors—was in fact overwhelming. Many of the registers were simply made up of data copied from other registers, meeting the reporting requirements of the many health programs operated through the ASHA program. These data, collected by ASHAs and collated at district, state, and national levels, were used to track targets and evaluate programs.

The paperwork ASHAs did was so complicated that it was hard for us to document in any straightforward way—it was part of many different programs of work, many different reporting streams, duplicated in several ways, and these systems were constantly changing. The various apps and mHealth initiatives that were adopted during the course of our fieldwork, whose stated goal was to streamline these operations, in fact made them more complex. Workers still kept all of the records on paper, and in addition also had to enter data into multiple apps.

"Enter Some Numbers and Give the Poor Woman a Rest!"

ASHAs found ways to make this extraordinarily burdensome data collection manageable. Like Kavita, who skipped weighing obviously healthy babies and simply noted down some number that seemed reasonable, many ASHAs skipped onerous data collection tasks with no clear connection to patient wellbeing, and they recorded some roughly appropriate figure instead.

Several scholars have noted that global health programs frequently have data requirements that are impossible for workers to manage without engaging in data fabrication. Patricia Kingori and Rene Gerrets have written about survey research expectations that are "unimplementable in practice" without the people collecting the data making "experience-based modifications."[2] Cal Biruk has pointed out that "genres of audit present themselves as technical transparency but embed submerged racialized suspicion"— underlying the desire for all this data is an inherent distrust that frontline workers are in fact doing their jobs.[3] But demands for yet more data may end up undermining the very care that data collection is designed to promote.[4]

When a new smartphone app for Anganwadi Workers was rolled out, ASHAs and Anganwadi Workers quickly found ways to bypass its incessant data collection alerts, entering in numbers to calm the app's notifications. The loading page for data entry on the app had an animation of a woman in a sari in motion. "Look at that poor running ASHA," an Anganwadi Worker commented as she input what she thought were roughly accurate figures in response to the app's many demands for data. "Enter some numbers and give the poor woman a rest!"

As in the meeting in the last chapter, where ASHAs were berated for incorrect data that was officially not their responsibility to collect, supervisors continually pushed ASHAs for more and more data. ASHAs resisted those demands. Sometimes the resistance was explicit, as in the ASHA who declared at the meeting, "We won't fill the register, it's not our job!" Sometimes the resistance was quieter, as in the Anganwadi Worker's making up numbers to give the poor running ASHA on the app a break.[5]

The ASHAs framed this resistance in both pragmatic and moral terms. Pragmatically, at the end of the day, the data didn't matter much to care provision—it was for the most part not used by ASHAs or by the primary health system to serve patients, but fed upward to serve the reporting demands of the system. It was used to supervise and evaluate ASHAs, but not to support patient care. ASHAs knew this and acted accordingly.

The resistance was also moral. Patricia Kingori and Rene Gerrets show that data fabrication by fieldworkers in global health studies can be an act of defiance by workers "against institutions that inadequately reward or exploit them, or against perceived unfair or abusive 'bad bosses.'"[6] They point out that institutional policies and practices toward workers affect data quality. This was absolutely the case in the ASHA program; faced with very low pay, no job security, and stunningly voluminous data reporting requirements, ASHAs made choices about how to spend their time. Weighing healthy babies didn't make the list of priority tasks.

As Kingori and Gerrets also point out, ultimately these acts of data fabrication and resistance do little to change top-down, abusive systems.[7] But for ASHAs, they were a way to manage them. In fact, it seemed to us, as a practical matter, that given the volume and diversity of data collection and reporting demands, they had little choice. This is not to say that ASHAs were making up the majority of the data they submitted; much, probably most, of it was quite systematically and carefully collected. But, given the extreme inefficiency of the system, keeping all of it fully up to date was not practical.

After COVID, the ASHAs in Rajasthan were relieved of the responsibility of filling out Anganwadi Worker registers. But that was in part because their work was growing in other ways.

Technology and Additional Work

While we were visiting with Bharti in 2023, she had to stop talking to us because her supervisors were calling her about Chiranjeevi Yojanā cards. Chiranjeevi Yojanā (literally, the Long Life Program) was a new health insurance program.

It was creating a lot of work for ASHAs. When we visited Kavita a few weeks later, she told us about it.

> Now they have put pressure on us to make the Chiranjeevi cards. "Make fifty of them every day." Nobody can make fifty cards in a day! Not more than ten or fifteen. Because there are problems with the network. And then all of the data has to line up in ways that aren't always possible. Sometimes a woman's mobile number isn't the one that is listed on her *aadhaar* card. Or someone's SIM card isn't working. Or someone else's SIM card is lost. Chasing after all of this, even ten or fifteen cards in a day is difficult.
>
> But the pressure is on for me to make fifty cards, every day. How can I do it?

This new card, as well as most of the other paperwork that ASHAs did, was now supposed to be entered into a new app. The new app, theoretically designed to make life easier for ASHAs, was making their lives very complicated. Every time an ASHA updated the app with information about one of their clients, that client would also get a notification. Often, that person would then call the ASHA to ask about it. This turned data entry into a social exercise that required an enormous amount of time. And, the government hadn't yet provided ASHAs in Rajasthan with smartphones, so sometimes they had to borrow phones from male family members to get the work done. Some ASHAs we worked with had smartphones of their own. In other families, only men had them. Bharti didn't have one yet.

Bharti was hopeful about the phones though—the newspapers had said that *all* women in Rajasthan were going to be given smartphones by the government. "We're women! So if the government is going to give us a mobile phone, wonderful. We're not going to be able to get one any other way."

But the app had not eliminated paper records. It had just added another layer of work. Globally, the shift to "mHealth" for Community Health Workers has had complex effects, sometimes increasing flexibility but at other times creating more administrative tasks.[8] Bharti now had to fill out registers on paper *and* on the app. After she explained the app to us, Bharti went inside her house and brought out a pile of registers. "Just look at how much work there is!" she exclaimed.

A Day with the Snake Oil Salesmen

Because people valued the work that ASHAs and Anganwadi Workers did for them, their reach and trust within Gurha Sajjanpura was exceptional— likely stronger than any other group in town. This was illustrated for us in a surprising way by the tactics of some traveling salespeople.

One morning in 2019, we showed up at an Anganwadi Center to find the ASHA annoyed with some calls lighting up her phone. "Because we are so well connected in the village," the ASHA explained, "a lot of people want to use us to sell things." A traveling sanitary pad saleswoman, she reported, was trying to get her to act as an intermediary. She wasn't interested.

Later in the morning, the traveling salespeople in question showed up. They were a sharply dressed man and woman, both wearing blue. The woman was wearing a shirt and pants, something that marked her as from the city. Their pitch was smooth. "We're an MNC—multinational corporation—we have many products—but we're here for health. Education and health." They continued their spiel for almost an hour, mostly ignored by the Anganwadi Worker and the ASHA. They pushed the women to sell sanitary pads, to little effect, and left unrewarded.

Later in the day, we ran into the pair again at another Anganwadi Center. This time, they attempted to use Surendra, a reluctant participant, in a dynamic presentation of the virtues of a metal bracelet that would save Surendra from the radiation from his cell phone, magically improving his health. The ASHA, bored, fanned herself and Svea with a laminated work schedule.

Later, the ASHA explained that she had been burned by such people before. Some tricksters had convinced her to collect money from the people she served in order to multiply it in an investment. People gave the ASHA the money; they trusted her completely. When the money disappeared, the ASHA was heartbroken—the trust she had worked so hard to build over years had been damaged. She was not going to make a similar mistake again.

That fraudsters and traveling salespeople consistently attempted to work through ASHAs illustrates something important about the trust ASHAs had built up across rural Rajasthan. There was no other network with the same reach and influence as the ASHAs—their services were valued, and they were trusted. Presumably, the ASHAs in Gurha Sajjanpura could have made a cut of the profits if they connected their clients with the traveling salespeople. Maybe, some ASHAs took advantage of these moneymaking opportunities. But this ASHA's previous bad experience had left her wary. She valued the trust she had built up in the community too much, she said, to jeopardize it in this way.

Data Work

We provide these arguably mundane vignettes of ASHA work in so much detail because we want to give a bit of the texture of daily work, and because we believe there is an important point here: ASHAs are not really primarily health workers, or at least not health workers in the sense of people whose primary job is to provide clinical care. Rather, ASHAs are primarily data workers. As the vignettes illustrate, their working days were consistently focused on data collection, organization, and on helping people with paperwork.

They are not alone in this among health workers. Across the world, health workers spend much of their time collecting and collating data—a topic that has garnered a lot of interest in medical anthropology. Several scholars have pointed out that health data allows people who never set foot in a health center to understand what is going on—or at least to feel they understand what is going on—from afar. This can empower technocrats while disempowering those with firsthand knowledge of on-the-ground realities.[9]

Anthropologists have also shown that programs can end up serving data, rather than data serving programs. The efforts of health workers are often directed toward improving data, rather than improving health.[10]

These critiques apply in this case—at least to a point. It is certainly the case that ASHAs spent much more time on documenting the provision of health services than on actually providing health services. All of the meetings of ASHAs we attended focused on data collection and reporting, and irregularities in data collection and reporting.

And the reporting of the data was the focus of their supervisors. "Once I was gone on a trip several hours away, to visit a religious leader, and my supervisor made me come back to the health post *that* day—just to submit my paperwork," Kavita told us. "They have such a *grip* on you!"

But the data the ASHAs collected did more than just empower technocrats by providing them with the data they needed to create reports on population health (although of course it did that): it *also* benefited the people that ASHAs served. The ASHAs' efforts to help women get identity cards, bank accounts, their *Mukhyamantree Rājśrī Yojanā* benefits was enormously important, and enormously appreciated. There were no other staff in the government system with the inclination or the time to provide this kind of assistance. Because the ASHAs enabled the transfer of significant financial benefits to the families that needed it most, they likely had very significant impacts on health and wellbeing—if not exactly in the way that had been envisioned by the ASHA programs' founders.

CHAPTER 3

We have Honorable Work, but That's All

Women's Labor in Rajasthan

A few days after we followed her doing her work, we went to Kavita's house to meet her family for the first time. Her house was lovely—among the nicest we saw in Gurha Sajjanpura. It was a little out of town, so there was space around it, and green fields. The house was freshly painted, and on coming through the doors, we entered a room with a tile floor, a flat screen TV, and a satellite box.

We sat on the couches in the room, along with Kavita and her father-in-law. Kavita's sister-in-law came in to greet us too and sat on the floor—the usual place for young married women, physically below the other family members. The fact that Kavita chose to sit on the couch was unusual and significant—an example of the self-confidence that the ASHA position had given her.

In the next room, a large piece of bright orange cloth with beautiful silver embroidery was stretched out over a large frame. This was Kavita's sister-in-law's work—all the women in the family contributed economically to the household. Her sister-in-law explained that what she earned for embroidery depended on the design—but she earned as much or more doing embroidery at home than Kavita did working as an ASHA.

"We also work in the fields, we tend to the cattle, it's not as if I am only working as an ASHA," Kavita explained.

"There's so much work to do for the ASHA position," her father in law commented, "but they get almost nothing. *So* much work."

Her sister-in-law agreed: "If you look at the work she does, the money is nothing."

Empowered or Exploited?

Groundbreaking Indian CHW programs like the Jamkhed program managed to improve health in environments of scarcity, while simultaneously giving poor women a voice—or at least, this has been the narrative around these programs.[1] In the years since, a durable and prevalent discourse about women's empowerment and CHW programs has developed in glossy global health reports and slick websites. Globally, most CHW programs employ women; across the world, claims are often made that working as a CHW is empowering for the people in these roles.

It is worth examining these claims carefully. Whether these programs result in empowerment for the women who work in them is a complex question. The story in Gurha Sajjanpura is a case in point. Understanding "empowerment"—a word that has been so overused in global public health as to perhaps be meaningless—requires understanding the multifaceted power structures in women's lives.

Looking closely at ASHA work shows that it is deeply entangled with Rajasthani social structures. To understand these entanglements, first we have to talk about money. ASHA work is a job. And next, we will discuss honor, because ASHA work is a job that takes place in the context of rural Rajasthani society. Also, honor and pay are inextricably linked, in tricky ways.

"She Makes Nothing"

The amount women made as an ASHA, averaging less than $100 a month, was significantly less than these same women could have made by engaging in unskilled labor. Another ASHA explained her dissatisfaction with a recent very small wage increase: "Look, the raise we're getting now, compare that to people who work in the fields. Look at the difference in our wages. And they're uneducated. I think looking at our work, our salary should be proportional to that. But we don't get that."

The fact that these educated women were paid less than unskilled workers stung them. "An Anganwadi Worker should make at least Rs 10,000 [a month; about $150]," one Anganwadi Worker explained. "Because it shouldn't seem to her family members as if she isn't helping the family. Some of our families say, 'She just wastes the whole day' (*din bhar yūṅ hī kharāb kar dete hain*). A maid who works in other people's houses, she makes more than we do."

Like many CHWs across the world, ASHAs had a complicated relationship with their work; they were proud of what they did to help others, even as many were angry over what they saw as exploitation.[2] Nearly all spoke of the value of their work. They all also said that the low salary and their competing work responsibilities created stress.

Many ASHAs' families were also frustrated by the low pay. One family discussed this issue when we visited them at home:

> ASHAS' FATHER-IN-LAW: The salary is extremely low. This is a big problem. She has this huge bag full of work to do. Like a big officer! [laughing] But she makes nothing.
>
> HUSBAND: The salary, for as much as she works, it might as well be nothing. . . . Every month they ask for a survey, two or three times. Every week, one or two meetings. You have to go to Gurha Sajjanpura. Then you have to call women about vaccinations. They ask for the records. Then we also get angry. The pay is so low, and there's so much work. Why are we giving so much to them?
>
> MOTHER-IN-LAW: She makes so little money, and we are paying for day laborers to do her fieldwork.

The ASHAs' supervisors, too, were frustrated by the low pay. One commented, "Whoever works, they are working because they want to make money. Of course, this job is service to society. But women have responsibilities at home. They have children to provide for."

"You Are Going Out for Your Tiny Little Salary?"

COVID intensified all of these pressures. Because routine health services weren't happening, ASHAs stopped getting their incentive-based payments, drastically lowering ASHA salaries even as the work increased. There was a Corona supplement of Rs 1,000 ($12) a month, but it didn't make up for the lost incentive-based pay. "It was a big financial loss," Kavita explained. She elaborated:

The thing was, we wanted to stop working and stay at home. Everyone wanted that, at that time.

But, we also had a responsibility as an ASHA. So I said, okay, let's serve the country. If I die, so what?

But my family told me not to go. They said, people who make two lakh rupees ($3,000) a month are sitting at home, and you are going to go out and put yourself at risk for your tiny little salary? But what to do? I also felt I had a duty. I had to go.

Still, my family was scared. Sometimes I was able to explain to them that look, I have a job to do. Other times they criticized me, and then I would just listen quietly.

Once the COVID pandemic passed, Kavita's salary went back to normal. But Kavita felt that the lessons of COVID had not really translated. "Even people in the government now appreciate our work more," she commented. "Nobody ever says anything against the ASHA. But at the same time, nobody says we should get a raise in pay. Nobody says it. Nobody."

Yet, few women left the ASHA position. To understand why, it's helpful to understand the social context of work in Gurha Sajjanpura more broadly.

"A Man's Salary Alone Isn't Enough to Support a Family"

It was not only ASHAs who engaged in wage work in addition to work in the home and fields: many of Gurha Sajjanpura's young married women did so. In a broader atmosphere of high unemployment and drought related to climate change, many ASHAs and other women said that it was impossible to rely only on agriculture and men's income. Some also mentioned the pressures created by social media to display status items like new clothing and store-bought birthday cakes. In the intensely social and status-conscious world of rural Rajasthan, these concerns were not frivolous; maintaining a solid social position had real impacts. "These days," one woman explained, "a man's salary alone isn't enough to support a family. So women are all working too."

Women in Rajasthan have traditionally sewed for others from their own homes and worked in the fields. These jobs were thus widely accepted as honorable and appropriate for young women. At the same time, they were also not aspirational: girls did not dream of doing embroidery or tending crops when they grew up. Doing sewing piecework usually earned women only a few thousand rupees per month; working in neighbors' fields paid Rs 250 per day.

Some other jobs for women carried social disapproval, an aura of being in desperate straits. Construction work, for example, was hard labor that paid Rs 300 to 350 per day for women (and Rs 400 to 600 per day for men). The government's MGNREGA (Mahatma Gandhi National Rural Employment Guarantee Act) program employed women to labor on public works projects for 195 rupees per day. Fully veiled women carrying large loads of construction materials were a common sight in Gurha Sajjanpura, but these jobs were not ones that educated women cared to take.

Instead, educated women aspired to jobs in education, healthcare, or government administration. Our respondents repeatedly referred to these as *izzat kī naukrī*—honorable jobs. These positions marked those who worked in them as modern and higher class, even as many workers still simultaneously desperately needed the income these jobs provided. We heard this phrase—*izzat kī naukrī*—again and again, from many women.

This was a concern they shared with many women across India. Indian women in work settings from beauty parlors to piecework are deeply concerned with honor and respectability, because these are important social factors with real material effects. Achieving a middle class, not lower class, persona is critical for many women.[3]

"What Choices Are There for a Woman?"

Women's education levels underwent a dramatic shift in Gurha Sajjanpura in the past generation. Twenty years ago, few women in rural Rajasthan were literate.[4] Most of the older Anganwadi Workers we spoke to—women in their forties—commented that when they were selected for the job twenty years ago, they had been recruited because they were one of the few educated women in town.

That dynamic has changed. As in other parts of North India, education is increasingly important for securing a good marriage for girls in Rajasthan.[5] Having educated daughters also positively affects the broader social status of the family.[6] Now, not only literacy, but higher education including graduate study, is common in Gurha Sajjanpura.

Higher education was a status symbol that could gain women marriage into a higher income, higher status family. But many women also wanted the years they had spent in school to actually go to use. "I'm educated, so there should be some use for that education," an Anganwadi Worker explained.

Thus honorable work—like ASHA work or other jobs that required education—was very attractive to women in Gurha Sajjanpura. They could make a little money; they could avoid engaging in stigmatized work; and they could put their education to use in the service of others.

Many ASHAs' families were deeply proud of the honorable work the ASHAs did. One ASHA's father-in-law, who himself had spent a lifetime as a construction laborer, commented:

> Her salary is low. But everyone in town, they tell me my daughter-in-law is so intelligent. When the doctor calls her in, she goes and works at the hospital. She's paid nothing, but what choices are there for a woman?
>
> She's educated, right? What is the point of being educated—if you can get government work, that's a huge benefit. Even if you just have a fourth class peon job, it's government work. The salary is low, but there's value in it. . . . When you wake up and know you have a job to go to, that is honorable work (*izzat to hai hi ki din uṭh ke dhanda milegā*).

This man compared the honorable work of a government job, where you wake up in the morning and can feel confident that your job exists, to the insecure and contingent work of day labor in fields or sewing (or the construction work he himself did). He took pride in his daughter-in-law's holding such a position—even though her pay was minimal.

The fact that ASHA work was honorable made it attractive even though the pay was very low. There were few honorable jobs available to women in Gurha Sajjanpura; most were accessible only to men. So women, despite their deep frustrations with the pay, tended to stay.

"We have Honorable Work—but That's All"

In contrast to most government jobs, ASHA work is contingent. Both ASHAs and Anganwadi Workers were "voluntary" workers, meaning that they earned less than minimum wage and did not enjoy the benefits or job security of "permanent" government employees. Scholars have noted that the voluntary status of Anganwadi Workers "can be seen as an illustration of the State's ability to violate its own labour regulatory framework, particularly in an arena such as care, where women are predominant."[7]

Women often mentioned a government job as a school teacher as the ideal honorable work: it was "permanent," meaning it included a substantial salary, job security, and benefits. Anganwadi Workers and ASHAs did not get such benefits.

ASHA work paid well below minimum wage. However, most other work for educated women in Gurha Sajjanpura was not much better. Many educated women, for example, worked for local private schools, and were paid around Rs 5,000–Rs 7,000 (about $80) per month.

This low wage was deeply gendered. Men with equivalent educational levels made much more—and had many more options. One young woman who worked as a teacher in a private school commented, "Even if they raise our pay, they'll raise men's more. They'll keep us at one level, and men at a higher level." Thus gender inequality in pay intersected with gendered ideas of honor in severely limiting job options for women in Gurha Sajjanpura.

It was precisely the honorable nature of the work—combined with gender inequality—that drove wages down to almost nothing. Maria Mies wrote of in-home lacemakers in rural India in the 1970s that the tenacity with which women clung to honorable work "even when they are virtually starving, is the ideological and psychological base on which a new phase of exploitation can be built up."[8]

Skilled work opportunities in rural Rajasthan were in short supply in general, and employment opportunities for educated women were particularly scarce. Because educated women preferred these jobs over manual labor, every honorable job for women was in extremely high demand. And honorable *government* jobs for women—even "voluntary" jobs like ASHA positions—were in the highest demand of all. These factors allowed remuneration to fall below poverty level wages. Almost all honorable jobs for women in town were extremely poorly paid.

ASHAs and Anganwadi Workers were not blind to the exploitative nature of their jobs. It rankled. While they were proud of what they did to help others, many of these women were angry. One ASHA bitterly commented, "we have honorable work—but that's all" [*Bas yah hai ki izzat kī naukrī le ke bhete hain*].

"People Like Us, We Get Ground Up and Spit Out"

Women and their families hoped that eventually, ASHA work would become "permanent"—a government job with tenure, pay and benefits, like other jobs in government schools and government health centers. This was the central reason the women stayed in their jobs, the central reason they were studying via correspondence courses: if permanent work became an option, they wanted to be ready for any potential educational requirements.

We heard about the desire for permanent work repeatedly, in nearly every interview. In the context of low pay, ASHAs and their families remarked again and again that they only reason they stayed in these jobs was because they hoped the jobs would become regular government employment. Often, an ASHA's mother-in-law and father-in-law—ultimately responsible for deciding labor allocation within the family—would encourage her to stay in the job, citing potential long term benefits. One father-in-law's discussion of this issue was typical:

> What she's getting now, it's basically nothing. . . . Sometimes I get angry, I say she should just quit this job (*golī lagāo*). She gets stressed. We get stressed. And we think, it doesn't make any sense to be doing this. But then I think, who knows, what will happen in the future? If she becomes permanent, she can earn a living, right from here. . . . You have to believe that will happen (*viśvāsa hī to karanā hai*), otherwise there's too much work in this job, it makes no sense.

One Anganwadi Worker discussed the issue with her husband, who was a government teacher:

> HUSBAND: So the teaching that I do, I get 80,000 rupees [per month] for it. And she gets 7,000.
> ANGANWADI WORKER: And I have more work than he has.
> HUSBAND: She has so much work. The government wants to raise their salaries, but it's not able to. . . . There are so many of them [Anganwadi Workers], making them all permanent is a huge financial commitment. When the Anganwadi program started, nobody was thinking that the government could ever make them permanent. But now, a lot of people are thinking that.

There was some precedent for this hopeful thinking. There was a pattern in Rajasthan in which cadres of government workers who had endured very low pay for years eventually became permanent. Parateachers in the school system had become permanent after nearly a decade; ANMs in the health system had become permanent after many years of voluntary work; the people who dug holes for electrical poles, too, had endured years of low pay and were ultimately rewarded with a permanent job.

Over time, shifts in the ASHA program had increased workers' hopes that they would eventually become permanent workers. First, there had been enormous increases in the work burden. Also, with time, more educated women from more powerful, politically connected families had begun taking these jobs.

At the same time, permanence was not a foregone conclusion for ASHAs and Anganwadi Workers. Many of them told us that Maneka Gandhi, a national-level minister, had said some years ago that Anganwadi Workers should become permanent. However, we could not find this quote; we did find repeated instances of Gandhi saying that making Anganwadi Workers permanent employees was "not possible" given the budget she had to work with. At the state and national levels, there was not a consistent enthusiasm for regularizing these huge cadres of workers; it was simply extraordinarily expensive to do, and some government stakeholders were not convinced it would pay off.[9] A very few ASHAs and Anganwadi Workers were able to gain permanent jobs by being promoted to supervisory positions; but most spent their careers waiting.

They said that they were "stuck"—if the jobs ever became permanent, they needed to stay in their positions when that happened. And, there were few better options: with the exception of government teachers, nearly all the honorable jobs for women in Gurha Sajjanpura were similarly low paying.

What ASHAs and Anganwadi Workers did receive were a series of very small raises. This was something, but most commented that it was not enough. "We've heard that it will happen, we'll become permanent," one ASHA said. "Right now, they're giving us a raise, but I'd rather not get that—instead give us benefits. Today I can work, I'm able bodied. But when I get old, and am forced to retire, what will I get then (*kis cīz ke sahāre jīenge*)?"

This ASHAs' concerns were quite valid. We visited one retired Anganwadi Worker who had no retirement benefits at all, and she bitterly recounted how she gave the best years of her life to the program, only to be left with nothing once she retired.

"This isn't retirement!" she cried. "They threw me out!" Both she and her husband were frankly angry:

FORMER ANGANWADI WORKER: I was thinking, "Okay fine, I'm a temporary worker. I don't make much. But in the future, I'll become permanent. I'll get more money." Believing that, I ruined my life (*bharose hī bharose mẽ jīndagī kharāb kar lī*).

HUSBAND: This is exploitation. The ones who sit in offices, they don't do anything. They don't work at all. They get all the benefits. And the temporary workers, they do everything. *Cakkī mẽ pīs rahe haiṅ, yah sab.* People like us, we get ground up and spit out.

Honor and CHW Work

As Padmini Swaminathan points out, employing ASHAs under contracts that violate the state's own labor laws both creates and perpetuates gender inequality.[10] The "voluntary" government jobs in Gurha Sajjanpura—ASHAs, Anganwadi Workers, Anganwadi Helpers, and material workers—were overwhelmingly female. By providing honorable work, and keeping the mirage of permanent employment in view but always just out of reach, the Indian state has, perhaps unintentionally, created a system that exploits the labor of over two million women.

Women in Gurha Sajjanpura, like women everywhere, did their best to make the most of themselves and their lives within the paths available to them. Within the clear path laid out for them across each stage of their life cycle, they tried to make an impact. The path of becoming an ASHA was attractive to many women because of what it represented: honorable work, the chance to make a difference in the community, the potential of someday having a permanent government job. But increasingly, women found that the permanent job was unlikely to happen soon, and the wages were obviously exploitative. The ASHA path proved deeply disappointing for many. But in the absence of other workable job options, they were stuck.

Yet these women saw more transformative possibilities on the horizon—or at least, they hoped for them. They valued the knowledge and the space their work provided, one outside the structures of their families. And they looked forward to a day when their work was rewarded with the salary and benefits they deserved.

It is a bit tough to know how realistic this aspiration of stable, minimum-wage work was. The policymakers we spoke to nearly all said that converting millions of ASHAs and Anganwadi Workers, not to mention the lower-status Anganwadi Helpers, into permanent government jobs was somewhere between unlikely and impossible.

Yet the dream of becoming permanent government workers was robust for all of the ASHAs and Anganwadi Workers we knew, as well as their families. If that happened, an Anganwadi Worker commented sardonically, "we could leave the cows behind and focus on *this* work."

"Then," an ASHA said, "we could actually make something of ourselves."

CHAPTER 4

If There's No Problem at Home, There Will Be No Problem Outside

Shifts in Family Structures

We had been following Anju in her work for a while before we met her family. We had visited with her when she spent time at her small, bright Anganwadi Center. We had gone with her door-to-door for her ASHA work, where we watched her patiently and cheerfully help poor women from nomadic families access critical government benefits. We even saw her lend small amounts of money to impoverished women to help them get paperwork filed.

Across all these interactions, Anju radiated a friendly, quiet competence. She was softspoken, but she was confident. And she crossed social barriers easily.

The nomadic families that lived in Anju's catchment area lived literally and figuratively on the margins of society in Gurha Sajjanpura. Many of them lived out of wagons (fig. 4.1). When those people went to weddings or other events in town, they stayed on the margins, not sitting in the company of others. For a woman from an impoverished nomadic lower-caste family, speaking to Anju, an educated woman from an established family, would normally be hard to do. Yet we watched Anju move through the neighborhood comfortably, being greeted warmly and answering bureaucratic questions with an approachable confidence.

Anju explained to us how she found value in this work:

> At first I really wanted to quit. It was so hard. . . . At that time I didn't know anything. I had never worked outside the house. I'd never written up a report. It was so, so, difficult.
>
> I didn't know anybody. And I worried so much about *ghūṅghaṭa* [the veiling and seclusion expected of young married women].
>
> But now? I can talk to anybody. I know about everything, right? It was hard then. But it's no problem now. I do all my work easily. And I get respect from everyone in town.
>
> And, it's so satisfying, making sure no child misses their immunizations. And that women are taken care of when they are pregnant. And helping out with malnourished children, helping their parents understand what to feed them.

So, we had gotten to understand Anju and her work. But the more we followed Anju—and other ASHAs—the more we realized that without talking to their families, we were missing a key part of their stories. For one, many ASHAs did not know the answers to the questions we asked them about why they had decided to become ASHAs in the first place. They hadn't decided, they explained to us. Their mothers- and fathers-in-law had decided. And they didn't know what had gone into that decision-making process.

Also, we were increasingly struck by how much freedom and mobility ASHAs had compared to other young women in Gurha Sajjanpura. Anju, for example, zipped around town on a *scooti*—a small motor scooter. This was definitely not common for women in the area, and absolutely not for young women. Why had Anju's family decided to grant her that much freedom, freedom that would certainly expose the family to gossip? Again, Anju told us, that decision had been made by her mother- and father-in-law. To understand it, we would need to talk to them.

"It's Good to Have a Backup Plan"

When Anju took us to her house one day after work, Anju's father-in-law welcomed us into the unpainted cement home; we sat in a large, clean, and sparse room. Anju's mother-in-law entered with Anju's chubby nine month old baby, fresh from his bath. She dried him off as we chatted. Anju's husband was away at work in town, but that hardly mattered; these people, her mother- and father-in-law, were the ones who had made the decisions about Anju's work and mobility.

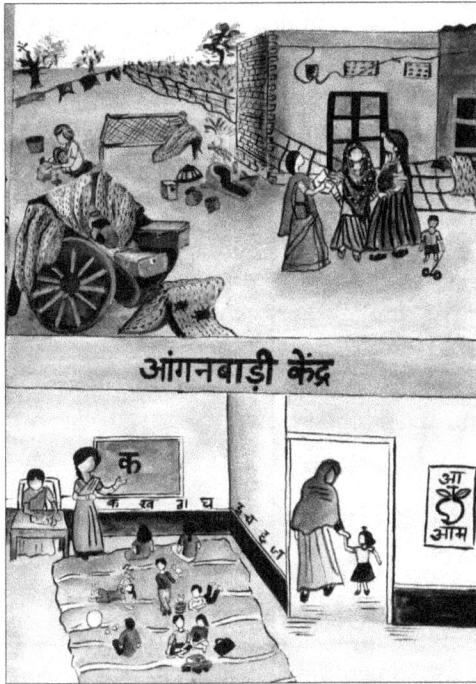

Figure 4.1. Anju at work. In the top panel, she fills out paperwork for a nomadic family. Below, she helps out in the Anganwadi Center, a preschool child care and nutrition center. Illustration © Soniya Kanwar.

When we mentioned what Anju had told us earlier, that she was thinking of quitting at first, her father-in-law laughed.

> Yes, it's true. She was really ready to quit! I told her, you know, sometimes you have to go through difficult times to see good times. I told her, it's true you're paid very little, but if you're made a permanent government worker in the future, it will all be worth it. Then you'll have a government job with benefits, plus you'll have the security of our farm and fields. I told her, I put you in that job, and I'll support you in it.
>
> Otherwise, she would have quit. There is so much work, and the money is so bad. But if she becomes a permanent government worker, if she makes five or ten thousand rupees a month, she'll be set up for life.

"There's no water in the ground anymore," Anju's mother-in-law added. "It's good to have a backup plan, not just depend on agriculture."

This, it turned out, was a common theme among the families we spoke to.

The economic changes happening in rural Rajasthan were far-ranging and swift. Farming—which had been the economic bedrock of rural Rajasthani society for many hundreds of years—was becoming increasingly unreliable due to climate change and dwindling water availability. Higher education, including for women, was opening up new options, but it was not clear which of those options would be economically viable in the long term. Within the family as an overall economic unit, it made sense to diversify: to deploy the labor of young family members in a variety of jobs, in the hopes that some would pan out. Putting your daughter-in-law in an ASHA job was a calculated bet: if the job became a permanent government position, that would ultimately be good for the family, and so it was worth a significant investment of time and support now.

"There Was No Cheating, and Our Team Won"

Because honorable government jobs for young women were in such high demand, obtaining a post as an ASHA or Anganwadi Worker was difficult. Navigating the complex politics and paperwork of getting an ASHA or Anganwadi position was not something that young married women could typically do alone. In Anju's case, as in most others, the process of obtaining one of these jobs was initiated and managed by the woman's family, generally her father-in-law.

Families often began working their connections in an attempt to secure their daughters-in-law ASHA and Anganwadi positions even before those posts became officially available. For example, when rumors began that an Anganwadi post would open up, Gurha Sajjanpura's *sarpanch* (the elected leader of the *gram panchayat*) received calls from a number of families on behalf of their daughters-in-law; some offered bribes.

A particularly politically savvy ASHA named Anita explained to us how this all worked:

> ANITA: These days, people really want ASHA posts. They're ready to give a bribe of one or two lakh rupees ($1,200–$2,500).
> SVEA: Why are they doing that, when the work is so hard, and the pay so low?
> ANITA: Most people aren't really aware how much work is involved, they think we just wander around doing nothing. . . . They think: if I spend one or two lakh rupees now, I'll get a job for life! Or at least, I'll be on the

track to a job for life, God or the government might make it permanent someday. They think, they should get a seat on the train, then if it ever actually leaves the station they'll be on it!

But even for politically connected older men, the process of obtaining an ASHA or Anganwadi position for their daughters-in-law could be challenging. Selection happened through a complex process. On one side, there were the official requirements, including educational requirements, of the Ministries of Health and Women's Affairs. But, the process also involved the *gram panchayat,* a local council of elected leaders. Thus political dynamics as well as the formal educational requirements played into ASHA and Anganwadi Worker selection.

One man who was a *ward panch*—an elected member of the *gram panchayat*—described the process of getting his daughter-in-law into an ASHA position. First, he explained his desire to get employment for her in the context of limited options. "She really wanted to do it, and she worked so hard on her education. And she's very responsible," he explained. "So we think, what can we do?"

But getting an ASHA position, he explained, "is very difficult. Nowadays, if there's one seat open, there are fifty applications for it. And the priority goes to the educated ones." So in addition to filing the necessary paperwork with the relevant ministry officials, he assembled a "team" to support his daughter-in-law's application at the *gram panchayat*. He lobbied the others in the group, in one case asking the wife of an elected official to make his case. "We did the work properly, there was no cheating," he explained. "And our team won!"

But even once his daughter-in-law had secured the appointment, there were additional barriers. The previous ASHA—who had been removed from the position by the government because she had reached the mandatory retirement age of sixty—did not want to give up the post.

"The previous ASHA's family blamed me," he explained, "saying, 'you kicked her out of the ASHA position' (*āpane usako haṭā diyā*). So I went to their house. In the end, they accepted it (*vah śānt huī*)."

Such controversy over ASHA and Anganwadi Worker positions was common. In another instance, the family of a young woman who had been passed over for an open Anganwadi Worker position filed a court case alleging inappropriate political interference—and won. As one of our interviewees told the story, the politically connected young woman was removed from the Anganwadi post, and the more educated woman got the job.

But another interviewee told it differently. In *her* telling, it was the *original* Anganwadi Worker who had been chosen through the correct bureaucratic channels, and the court case was a ploy to get the politically powerful family's choice into the position. "Whoever is powerful, they'll get it. Whoever has a strong stick will own the buffalo," this woman said.

Whichever version of this story is accurate—and both probably held some truth—what was clear was that selection for these positions was political and contested, and that families jockeyed to get their daughters-in-law into these positions.

"The Person Who Doesn't Need It, Don't Give It to Them!"

The politics of ASHA selection were shaped by political connections. But they were also shaped by morals and optics. The *gram panchayat* couldn't repeatedly choose politically connected women to be ASHAs—they also had to consider how those selections would be perceived among their constituents more broadly. Thus both political connections (generally favoring wealthier women) and the need for the job (generally favoring poorer, more marginalized women) could play into the selection of an ASHA, at different ways in different times. Anita explained:

> The *sarpanch* used to be able to just select someone, but not now. People are aware of the value of an ASHA job, and there is political pressure to give it to a woman who needs the money.
>
> People say, the person who doesn't need it, don't give it to them! Like, if a woman has a twelfth-grade education, but her father-in-law is a headmaster and her husband is a teacher, then she doesn't need the ASHA job. Instead, it should be given to a widow, someone trying to raise her children alone. She really *needs* the post.
>
> Sometimes, the *gram sabah* might have someone more qualified, but they also look at people's family situations, who needs the job more. They might give it to someone who has a desperate need for even the three to four thousand ($50) a month she would get as an ASHA. So then the *sarpanch* might go explain to the more educated woman: "What will you do with that ASHA job? You have a BA, you should go teach in a private school, you might make a few thousand more. Or, study a bit more and get a higher level job. The ASHA job has nothing in it for you."

Optics were complex not just for selection—they also played out after ASHAs were chosen. Having drawn on connections to get their daughters-in-law selected for ASHA and Anganwadi Worker positions, families also experienced social pressure to ensure that these women performed their jobs well. Once his daughter-in-law started work as an ASHA, the *ward panch* quoted above found that the position presented challenges for her:

> There was a time when my daughter-in-law wanted to quit, although she didn't say so directly. She was so worried [about the workload]. I told her, if you quit, it's no problem, it's not as if you're earning anything from it. 500 rupees or 800 rupees, whatever.
>
> But, if she doesn't do good work, people will complain about us and our family. They'll say she was appointed because of political connections but doesn't do anything.

He explained that ultimately, his daughter-in-law decided to stay in the job, but the family cut back on her responsibilities at home in order to make her workload reasonable and ensure that she could carry out her ASHA duties to the best of her ability.

"We Are Paying for Day Laborers to Do Her Fieldwork"

The *ward panch* was not alone in making significant sacrifices in order to keep his daughter-in-law in the ASHA job. Once they got the job, ASHAs generally found it challenging, and families discovered that they needed to make significant changes to the structure of the family's work in order to free up time for the daughter-in-law to work as an ASHA.

Anju's family discussed this with us too. They said that keeping Anju in the ASHA job was hard on the family. "It costs us a lot of money to help her do the work," her father-in-law commented, "so it all adds up to nothing in the end."

The lost labor to the family was significant—Anju spent many hours a day at work as an ASHA, time that she otherwise would have spent doing fieldwork at home. Her father-in-law sometimes hired day laborers to make up that work; each one cost the family Rs 250 per day, plus tea, plus transport—much more than Anju made through her ASHA work.

Like Anju's family, many families hired help to do the fieldwork that their daughter-in-law could not. Many families incurred significant costs in supporting an ASHA or Anganwadi Worker, from paying for transport to replacing the woman's labor.

Families also took on responsibility for ASHAs' and Anganwadi Workers' extensive work at home, cooking and caring for her children. Those tasks generally fell to the ASHAs' sisters-in-law and mothers-in-law.

In cases where families were not willing to make such accommodations, women found it hard to hold onto ASHA or Anganwadi positions. For example, one ASHA said that her predecessor had to quit. "She couldn't do the door-to-door work [of the ASHA position]," she explained. "Her mother-in-law, her father-in-law, her husband, they didn't support her. So, she was forced to quit (*majbūrī mẽ choṛnā paṛ gayā*)."

ASHA work significantly shifted work relationships at home. Families made profound changes in the division of labor. Mothers- and fathers-in-law deployed the labor of other family members—or of paid help—to make up for the agricultural work and housework the ASHA could no longer do. These shifts are striking because they illustrate the deep flexibility and pragmatism of Rajasthani households. Despite the strict structure and hierarchy of the rural Rajasthani family, the need to ensure financial stability in the context of social and climate change meant that the older generation that held control in these families were willing to significantly alter the traditional division of labor in order to support ASHAs in their work. One of the most significant shifts was in young women's mobility.

"A Lady Driving a Scooti!"

Anju's house was several kilometers from the Anganwadi Center, and several more from the health center where Anju filed her reports. To avoid having a young woman walking these distances alone, her father-in-law walked with her at first. But this, too, was an issue: it took up a great deal of his time, and both of them were exhausted from walking so far in the brutal heat of the Rajasthani summer. Anju's mother-in-law worried about both of them.

So, in a move nearly unheard of for young women in this area, Anju's in-laws decided to buy her a *scooti*, or a small motor scooter. Now, Anju drove around the village, veiled and confident, covering the long distances she needed to travel—to do her fieldwork, to file paperwork, to get from her house the health center—quickly and easily. Yet this, too, cost money: Anju's entire ASHA salary went toward the *scooti* loan payment and the Rs 300 per month it cost to keep the *scooti* fueled.

Anju's path to *scooti* ownership had been paved by other women in town. The first woman to ride a *scooti* in Sajjanpura was an Anganwadi Worker, a woman who had been with the program almost since its inception and who was among the first women in Sajjanpura to hold a government position.

"Before, in the village, no women used a scooti," her husband explained. "When people saw her, they were surprised: a lady driving a scooti! But in Rajasthan, it's like this: once one person has gone down a road, others will follow (*eka ko dekh ke dūsara usī rāste par chalte hain*)."

He was right: the groundbreaking and socially risky move that his wife took in riding a *scooti* had ripple effects. Because of the substantial work involved for men in supporting an ASHA's mobility, *scootis* were seen as a reasonable investment by many families. Without one, families had to invest a huge amount of male labor in escorting the ASHA from place to place. Another ASHA's husband explained:

> HUSBAND: The thing is, I am busy myself. She doesn't make enough for someone else to spend all of their time supporting her (*uske lie piche piche kar din*). And look, we have a lot of work in the fields. You lose all kinds of work time bringing her there, bringing her back. . . . That's why it became necessary to get her a *scooti*.
>
> SURENDRA: Did people react negatively to her using a *scooti*?
>
> HUSBAND: At first when we got the *scooti*, people in the village had issues. But when she walked, some people also had negative thoughts. Anyway, as she kept doing it, people stopped thinking about it. They moved on to other things.

Family support for ASHA mobility was particularly critical in the early stages of employment. Training involved travel to another city, a task that was well beyond the experience of many young women. This could add up to weeks of commitment from male relatives. One ASHA's father-in-law and sister-in-law discussed this:

> FATHER-IN-LAW: Then she had training. I went with her. Her baby girl was small, we left her behind. The baby was still being breastfed.
>
> SISTER-IN-LAW: The baby was only four or five months old, and [the ASHA] was gone for ten days. I fed her from a bottle. Then the younger baby, she was only fifteen days or a month old, when [the ASHA] started working. She would be gone from seven until noon. It's a lot of work! [*laughing*]

FATHER-IN-LAW: The mother-in-law, the sister-in-law, they do the work. You have to work.

SISTER-IN-LAW: Now, she has three kids, and they are my responsibility during the day. I look after them.

FATHER-IN-LAW: Now, [the ASHA] goes to the Anganwadi Center herself. But before, I had to bring her there to drop her off. It was difficult at first, but you know what? Now [the ASHA] goes to the district capital, she even goes to Jaipur by herself!

Like this father-in-law, many ASHAs' families took real pride in the ASHAs' expanding mobility, commenting on the sophistication and competence of their daughters-in-law. These shifts in mobility were truly notable, not only to us but also to ASHAs' families and to ASHAs themselves.

ASHAs' worlds expanded in profound ways, and what is particularly striking is that the very families that had previously enforced their seclusion *supported* them in expanding their mobility not only outside the walls of the house, but even to faraway cities. The potential for an ASHA to make long-term economic contributions to the family was enough for that family to dramatically widen her world.

But, ASHAs still lived in rural Rajasthan. This expanded mobility opened them up to gossip and community censure. Here, too, their families were key supporters.

"If There's No Problem at Home, There Will Be No Problem Outside"

We asked Anju's mother- and father-in-law about Anju's concerns about *ghunghat,* the system of seclusion that keeps many young married women in Gurha Sajjanpura at home. We wondered if they faced censure from others for allowing Anju to leave the house.

MOTHER-IN-LAW: Lots of people said things.

FATHER-IN-LAW: And they still do! They say, what's going on with her? She's just wandering here and there.

MOTHER-IN-LAW: They disrespect her, say she's going all over town, *raṇḍ roṭī phiratī hai.*

FATHER-IN-LAW: But what to say, if she gets a permanent government job, it will all be worth it.

MOTHER-IN-LAW: And you know what? Those same people come to us asking for help getting *their* daughters-in-law into that job. They ask us to tell them if any positions open up at the Anganwadi Center!

In rural Rajasthan, gossip about young women's mobility was gossip about morals. What is striking is that Anju never heard these rumors or objections. Instead, her mother- and father-in-law heard them.

Neighbors often voiced objections to an ASHA's mobility to the ASHA's family rather than the ASHA herself, the implication being that the young woman's mobility should be restricted for the good of the household. It fell to family members to protect and defend the young woman's mobility; when these defenses came from powerful elder family members, they were generally respected by neighbors.

One Anganwadi Worker's father-in-law talked about how he forcefully countered gossip: "There are some people who will say, '*Are yāra*, she went here, she went there. Today she went to Jaipur.' *Are*, of course she has a job, so she'll go! She'll go for work, and am I supposed to follow her around everywhere? She has work there, she'll go there. . . . The person who leaves their home, that person will understand the world."

Many families and young women alike commented on how, over time, ASHAs and Anganwadi workers experienced a revolutionary change in mobility. Another family discussed this issue:

ASHA'S HUSBAND: She [the ASHA] goes to [a nearby city] herself now! She used to be afraid, but now she goes out.
SVEA: What was she afraid of?
FEMALE FAMILY MEMBER: You worry about what people will say about you: Why is she going to other people's houses? What is the reason? People say lots of things like that.
FEMALE FAMILY MEMBER: If you go to an unfamiliar house, there may be a man there, how will he behave (*uskā kyā soc hogī*)?
HUSBAND: But now, everyone knows the ASHAs.
ASHA: Anyway, there's no problem in doing the work. If there's no problem at home, there will be no problem outside.

Women whose families did not provide such support found themselves facing intense conflicting pressures: pressure from their supervisors to get work done, and pressure from their families not to leave the house. Some supervisors were sympathetic to these issues.

Discussing the case of an ASHA who frequently failed to show up for work, one supervisor commented: "She has family problems that make it hard to work. Sometimes she just has to leave. Some people's families don't allow them out of the house. You know, some families, they put their daughters in law in these positions, and then they don't give them enough time to do the work."

In such cases, ASHAs generally did not last long at the job. For the most part, we were struck by how flexible families were in supporting their daughters-in-law.

Like Anju, many ASHAs considered quitting soon after they began work, both because of the low pay, and because of the stress that moving around the village independently caused them. Pay never ceased to be an issue. The mobility, on the other hand, came to be something that they valued greatly.

"I'm Not Dependent on Anyone"

For some ASHAs, the post also gave them another new freedom: control over a bit of money. How much control they gained varied depending on their family situation.

For families like Anju's, with substantial fields and other assets, the expense of keeping an ASHA or Anganwadi Worker in her job could be more than her salary. But for some other families living closer to the edge, without agriculture to support them, even the very low salary could bolster the family finances. An Anganwadi Worker's husband commented:

> We used to have water at the house, but now only seasonally, so we can't always grow things. So I do construction work too, when I can get it. I don't have a fixed job to run the family.
>
> So her job is helpful, right? When she gets six thousand [rupees per month], I bring in six or seven thousand, together we can make it fourteen or fifteen thousand. . . . So her job, it's a support. If she wasn't doing this, she'd have to go work in someone else's fields—she'd have to do something.

In some cases, as in this example, a woman's pay was pooled with the family finances. In other cases, women kept the money for their "own expenses" (*hāth kharca*)—usually clothes for themselves and their children, school fees and supplies for their children, and household items. For women whose finances were set up this way, it meant a lot not to have to ask for money from their husbands or in-laws for every purchase. An Anganwadi Worker commented, "It's good, from this work, I'm not dependent on anyone, I have my own spending money. Before, I had to be dependent on others."

The ability of a woman to control her own salary often depended on the overall financial health of the family. Another woman whose husband made almost nothing commented, "I give what I earn to my husband—some of it—I also spend some myself," but then added: "With only five to seven thousand [rupees per month for an ASHA salary; about $80], we can't ask our family to let us keep any for ourselves. If we were making more, then we could do something for our children."

Women who managed their finances separately from those of the family also found that the expenses involved in their work cut significantly into income. One ASHA commented:

> So what happens is this, sometimes they call me to the PHC [Primary Health Center], sometimes they call me somewhere else. Half of my salary gets spent on this. On going here and there. To get to my PHC, I have to walk, and then take a bus, and then walk again. If I get hungry somewhere along the way, I don't have a salary to pay for a snack.

Again and again, women commented that if ASHA work was better paid it would change their lives for the better, allowing them to justify their increased mobility to skeptical family members (there were a few of these in most families) and giving them more of their own cash to control.

"Even if it's a Small Job, It's Mine"

Some women gained a small measure of economic independence through their jobs. But more significant for many women was the broader independence. One woman discussed her emotions when she left her ASHA job in order to start a BA program:

> I was so sad. I even cried! It was so hard to sign my resignation papers. My husband said, "Why are you crying over 500 rupees? Take 500 rupees from me."
> I said, it's not about the 500 rupees, I went to the field, I got to know every-

body. And I earned it myself—even if it's a small job, it's mine. And everyone in the whole village had gotten to know me.

Many women described how leaving the house expanded their concepts of what was possible, both for themselves and for their daughters. They commented that it was practically helpful to be mobile: they could pick up items in the market or help family members navigate the hospital. They also talked about the relief of getting a few hours away from the extended family. "The pay is nothing—it disappears in one day," one ASHA explained. "But it's a way to get out of the house, and that helps me make it through (*is ke bahane bahar nikalte hain, to is mein hi sabr karte hain*)."

Other women whose home life was not happy noted that being an ASHA or Anganwadi Worker was a reprieve. "I go crazy at home (*dimākh bhī kharāb ho jātā hai ghar par*)!" one woman said, laughing. "We come here [to the Anganwadi center] and we can rest easy."

Shifts in Family Power Structures

Family structures bent to accommodate ASHA work; young women were provided with additional freedoms, and family members worked to support those freedoms. The availability of respectable government work for young women shifted family structures and women's lives in ways that were often profound.

Young women were often able to control a bit of money; they gained more freedom to move; they gained freedom from the constant supervision of their mothers-in-law; and with time, they gained understandings of the workings of the world beyond the walls of their home. These shifts occurred because of the potential—not yet realized—that ASHA work would lead to a secure, long-term income stream for the family. Family power structures bent because of hope: hope that investment in a young woman's capabilities would lead to the government rewarding those capabilities.

As they grew into their own, many ASHAs started to wonder if there was anything they could do within the ASHA program to advocate for a living wage. As those questions arose, some ASHAs, supported by their families, entered into a striking new chapter in their lives, one that would take them far from home.

CHAPTER 5

I'll Fight For Them

ASHAs as Leaders

Amid hundreds of women gathered at ASHA labor protests in the city of Jaipur, Anita stood out—she was always a center of attention and activity. Anita, in her late thirties, dressed plainly and did her hair simply. Outspoken and confident, she had a shimmering intellect. It was easy to get wrapped up in whatever Anita was saying—and she was usually saying it to a group of attentive women. We introduced ourselves and asked if she could make some time to talk with us.

On a hot summer afternoon, we drove several hours into the country-side to get to Anita's house. She welcomed us warmly and ushered us into the two dark small rooms where she lived. We sat on small wooden stools in one room, and looked around as she made tea in the other. Both rooms opened onto a dirt-floored courtyard open to the pale Rajasthani sky. We could hear the sounds of the other neighbors—a cough, murmured voices, a child's cry—through the crumbling brick walls, blackened from rain.

Anita's simple home reflected her modest financial situation. Her husband earned 12,000 rupees (about $150) a month, which Anita described as "nothing for savings, just enough to have food on the table." She said the money she made as an ASHA was an important support, and something that brought "balance" into the relationship between the two of them.

There was barely space for the three of us to sit in Anita's small room, but that all seemed to evaporate around us once Anita started talking— she was thoughtful, intelligent, funny, and shared with us a deep interest in the questions we were discussing. We sat and talked for several hours in the gathering dusk.

We can think of no more powerful way to tell Anita's story than in Anita's own words. Throughout this chapter, we include sections taken directly from what she told us. We translated her recorded words and edited for length and flow.

Anita's Story, I: "Wandering Around Like That Doesn't Look Good"

Years ago, shortly after I got married, someone told me there was an ASHA vacancy in my area, and I asked my father-in-law if I could apply. But he brushed me off, saying, "What will *you* do at the Anganwadi Center?"

You see, traditionally, people didn't allow women to work in those kinds of jobs. My father-in-law thought that work at the Anganwadi Center was *choṭī naukrī*—small work. These days, the big shots put their daughters-in-law to work at the Anganwadi Center! But at that time, they saw it as beneath them.

But I held onto the idea. Later, when I had a son, I said to my father-in-law, "All the women are getting work, so let me work too. If I work hard, ASHA work could lead to a government job in the end. And the work is just going from house to house visiting women. Anyway, they probably won't even hire me. So it really doesn't hurt to try."

But I was hired. I was hired, and then for the first two years I didn't do any work at all! I was hesitant to leave the home. Because here, there's a *ghūṅghaṭa* system. In going outside, *bahu*s, young women, they have problems.

And my family had problems too. They said, "Coming and going, wandering around the whole village like that, it doesn't look good." So, for two years after I got trained, I sat at home.

Actually, it was the families of other ASHAs who convinced my family to let me work. There were four other women who had been hired—my husband's aunt was one of them. She said to my family, "What's the problem? I'm going with her, right? Nobody is going to kidnap your *bahu!*"

So slowly, slowly I started going to a few meetings. I met the other women who had also been hired, and we used to gather together and then work together. The other women and I would tell each other, "You come with me and go door-to-door. And I'll go with you." Five of us would go in a group!

Bit by bit, I started to actually do fieldwork. We would all spend the day working on one woman's area. And the next day in another woman's area. We were all too afraid to do the work alone. But when we went in a group, the fear went away.

And then, in the end, we got to know the area. The shame dissipated, the fear dissolved. And we started to get to work.

Anita's Story, II: "I Thought, We Should Organize"

It was a few years later that I got involved in advocating for fair pay. There was a time when they raised pay for Anganwadi Workers, but not for us ASHAs. I had, like, a jealous feeling. I thought, we should organize.

Then I thought, I suppose I have to be a leader!

All the women I talked to said, "Let's go to Jaipur." If we were upset, ASHAs in other areas were upset too. Other women we reached out to said, "We'll go too." So we spread a fire in all of Rajasthan. In a field in Jaipur, fifty thousand ASHAs showed up to protest.

When we got there, I met Shiv Partap, the union leader. He heard me when I was giving a speech at the podium during the protest. He came to me, and he said, "If you can speak at a podium like that, you can definitely handle leading a union. Women will listen to you."

He said, "You make the union, and I'll guide it."

So in 2007, we joined him. He gave me control over one area. He gave another ASHA a different area. And organizing like that, dividing the areas among us, we created a union.

We found leaders for every district. Then, we organized women in each block [sub-district], and in each block we designated a leader. And we held protests, and they had effects. Through our action and protests, our 250 rupee salary became 500 rupees. Then we protested again, and we got 750. Then 1,000. Then 1,500. Then 1,600. And now, we get a 2,500 rupee salary. After doing all that work and fighting, we got to this level.

Without protests, that pay would not have been raised. Look, the government has found women who are willing to work for free! Without our activism, why would they change anything? If a baby doesn't cry, the mother doesn't feed it.

In addition to raises, we are saying that the path to becoming an

ANM should be open to ASHAs. Our responsibilities in pregnancy and delivery have multiplied. When there's no doctor, when the nurse is nowhere to be found, it's the ASHA who picks up the slack. So what if I haven't taken a course on childbirth—I have the practical experience! We know how these things work.

Shiv Partap supported me. He said, "She can hear women, and women can hear her. She has that quality of being able to listen to and sort out their problems."

Labor Unions in India

The union that Anita was part of was typical in India. India's labor movement was an influential part of the fight for independence against the British; when India gained independence, collective bargaining rules were established, and unions have held an important role in labor relations ever since. Often, unions agitate to ensure that employers operate according to Indian labor law.[1]

Most unions in India are affiliated with political parties.[2] In Rajasthan, the two biggest parties—which are also the two major parties in India as a whole—are the BJP (Bharatiya Janata Party, the party of the populist leader Narendra Modi) and the Congress party (Congress being the more left wing of the two). Both have ASHA unions. So does the communist party in Rajasthan, although unlike in some South Indian states, that party doesn't have much of a local following.

One result of the fact that each political party has its own union is that there are frequently multiple unions, affiliated with different political parties, attempting to represent the same workers. Because there isn't an established way to recognize one official union as representing workers in most sectors in India, each political party generally tries to recruit workers into their own union. And, in addition to unions affiliated with a given political party, there are also often independent unions, aiming to recruit workers who feel that the party-affiliated unions may not be effectively representing them.[3] This was the case with ASHA unions.

Anita's union was headed by a man named Shiv Partap. Shiv Partap was officially unaffiliated with any political party (although as we discuss further, he had extensive political ties and ambitions). But Anita never mentioned party ideology once in our hours-long interview. For her, the choice to affiliate with Shiv Partap was primarily practical, not ideological.

A Powerful Union Leader

One afternoon, we went to visit Shiv Partap. In addition to being a union leader, he also had a government job. When we reached his office—which was packed with people in rows of chairs across from a desk—we found Shiv Partap presiding at his desk in a crisply ironed peach colored *kurta pajama*. His forehead was marked with tika powder, a visible sign of his Hindu faith.

On the desk itself were stacks of worn papers bound in cardboard folders. A clerk came in and out to deliver papers; the clerk was visibly nervous in front of Shiv Partap, shaking as he handed over the files. Shiv Partap was a powerful and intimidating man.

Shiv Partap skillfully managed a stunning number of conversations and tasks at once: our interview, the papers he needed to sign for his bureaucratic position, what seemed to be nearly constant phone calls, and discussions with his political followers in the room. All of his stakeholders were simultaneously and artfully balanced.

Shiv Partap, between his other tasks and conversations, discussed the issues involved for ASHAs and Anganwadi Workers in a way that revealed his sophistication and his knowledge. He referenced the Labor Act in arguing that ASHAs should receive a minimum wage. He pointed out that at least thirteen other states had already raised the ASHAs' salary. He commented that in addition to the ASHAs' existing heavy workload, they were often assigned more tasks by their local *sarpanch.*

He explained what he saw as the role of the union. "If they ever have problems, if a supervisor comes down hard on them, then we are with them to solve the problem," he told us. "We made the union so that there can be power in numbers, so that all can be one."

Moving on to the question of permanent work, Shiv Partap again argued in passionate and compelling language that ASHAs, Anganwadi Workers and Anganwadi Helpers should have permanent jobs. He mentioned high-level national officials that he had met with to that end, and said he was disappointed that they had not followed through with action.

Shiv Partap's bureaucratic government job prevented him from having a formal party affiliation. But he was actively planning for when that job ended, and when he would join a party and perhaps run for office. Union organizing was a primary way he was gathering followers who he expected would support him in his political ambitions.

"He Started to Berate Us"

Meena, the woman whose story opens this book, was also a union leader. Her involvement in unions was how we had met her in the first place.

Several years ago, Meena explained to us, she had gotten tired of too much work for too little pay. She wanted to do something about it, and she saw labor unions as a way forward. She and some other ASHAs read in a newspaper that a union—Shiv Partap's union—was holding some rallies in Jaipur. Meena and her colleagues weren't members of the union, but they went to join the strikes anyway. A group of them got together, hired a bus, and went.

These strikes included not just ASHAs, Meena explained, but a range of government workers: electrical workers, roadway workers, Anganwadi Workers, sanitary workers. "There was just a huge crowd," Meena remembered. The women were gathered together, demanding fair pay.

Shortly after the strikes, the ASHAs' salaries were doubled, from Rs 500 to Rs 1,100 a month. Inflation ate much of the increase, but $20 a month was better than $10, and feeling that they had been a part of that change was energizing.

But the results were also somewhat disappointing: the Anganwadi Workers' salary was raised more than the ASHAs' salary was, leaving the ASHAs feeling a bit left behind. Meena and some other ASHAs went to complain to Shiv Partap. When they did that, Meena said, "He started to berate us. He said we hadn't been doing what he told us to do. A 500-rupee raise was plenty for us, he said."

Meena had been stewing over this when she met Shafique, the leader of a *different* union for ASHAs. He convinced Meena and her co-workers that he cared, that he would fight for them to become "permanent"—to get a real government job with salary and benefits, not a "voluntary" position with incentive payments. But this relationship too had been rocky. The women paid him 165 rupees (about $3) per year in union dues. Then, Meena explained, he asked for more money:

> He told us, "As well educated as you all are, with BAs and MAs, and with ten years of work experience, you should be made permanent. If they don't make you permanent in the ASHA job, they should give you another government job. I'm going to petition the courts for this, on your behalf. For this, I'll need 1,500 rupees (about $25) from each of you, for lawyers."

So I, all of us, we all gave him 1,500 rupees. This was a year ago. And so far, we have gotten nothing from it.

This situation was particularly tough for Meena, who had been the one to convince forty other women to chip in 1,500 rupees each—a large sum for these women, representing several weeks of work. Now that there was nothing to show for it, Meena faced blowback from the other women. They were upset: had Shafique tricked them into giving up badly needed, hard earned savings?

Gender and Labor Unions

The role that Anita and Meena played in their unions was typical of female activists in unions across India. Working women in many sectors participate in unions in India, and across contexts they tend to find that this opens new worlds to them: it expands their mobility, allows them to meet new people, lets them escape housework, and provides an opportunity to craft a public identity.[4] For the ASHAs we knew who were involved with unions, becoming an ASHA had first expanded their world. Then, joining a union expanded it further. Union leaders like Meena and Anita found their mobility and knowledge increased most of all. Both Meena and Anita traveled independently across Rajasthan, mobilizing women in their union roles.

Yet Meena and Anita were frustrated with their limited levels of power and voice within these unions. In India, many women find that, even as participating in unions expands their worlds, they are ultimately kept out of the highest leadership ranks of unions, which are dominated by men.[5] In the case of the ASHAs in Rajasthan, no union leader was an ASHA (and almost all of them were men). Women's participation can be limited by gender norms that discourage activities like travel, meeting with men, and attending meetings or protests at night (though Meena and Anita did all of these things). Women, too, can be more vulnerable to intimidation or harassment by their managers as a result of their union activities, especially as they have more limited options for other work.[6]

"She's the One Who's Always Running Off Her Mouth"

The ASHAs we knew who were union leaders—women like Meena and Anita—were extraordinary people. They had moved from the expectation that they stay secluded, to doing door-to-door to work as an ASHA, to traveling hundreds of miles and leading thousands of women in achieving social change. They did all of this with great intelligence, humor, and courage.

They did need courage, because being a union leader could be risky. Part of what Anita did on a regular basis was advocate for ASHAs that were being mistreated by their supervisors: verbally abused, denied the wages that were due them, or sexually harassed.

"If there is a problem for ASHAs at the Primary Health Center," Anita explained, "first we document the problem in writing, and if it isn't solved that way, then we give a warning. Like, 'This entire block of three hundred ASHAs will do a protest in front of your Primary Health Center.' This kind of work, that is how you sort out ASHAs' problems."

It was unfortunately not uncommon for ASHAs to experience harassment at the hands of supervisors, and for supervisors to deny them the pay they were due. Taking action in the way Anita did carried risk, because ASHAs faced potential retaliation for speaking up.

Group advocacy among ASHAs to solve problems was effective. It could also lead to consequences for the women who acted. An example here is Priya, an ASHA in a different village who was involved in unions but not an organizer. She discussed an ongoing situation in which the doctor at her health center was failing to submit ASHAs' paperwork to higher levels, leading to months of lost pay.

"When I complained," she said, mouth pressed into a thin line, "our supervisor told me the doctor is very politically connected." She continued:

> It's the person who complains who gets into trouble. But in my Primary Health Center, if someone is being mistreated, I can't watch that. I'll fight for them. Everyone else says, "I won't say anything." I say, "I'll speak up."
>
> But I knew I would get into trouble (*maiṃ hī burāī ke sāmne āūṃgī*). I knew that people would say about me, "Priya, she's the one who's always running off her mouth."
>
> Anyway, I brought it all forward to my supervisors. I said, "Look, if there are mistakes in my claim forms, then fire me, that's it. But I'm not going to put up with this harassment any more." That's what I said.

"My friend was right with me the whole time," Priya continued. Her friend was another ASHA. "Then the supervisor said to my friend, 'When you die, I'm going to throw your ashes into the Ganges.'"

Priya paused for a moment and we thought about how terrifying it must have been to hear this veiled threat. What the supervisor was saying here was that he could destroy this ASHA. Nothing concrete had happened, and Priya was determined not to give up.

Still, she was shaken: "Our supervisors in ICDS [Integrated Child Development Services, responsible for the Anganwadi Centers] berate us, the ones in the medical system berate us, we have nobody's support. We are twisting in the wind between them. One grabs one leg, one grabs the other. We're there in the middle, being pulled apart."

Anita, too, had experienced retaliation. Once, her supervisors cut three months of her salary. This cut into her ability to feed and clothe her family.

Still, union leadership also had benefits for leaders. Some got some paid for the time they spent on union work. They got respect from their peers. And they could feel that they were part of something bigger, part of pushing for justice. Anita and Meena both found the work exhausting, but both were also compelled to do it. Anita commented:

> Sometimes I get tired, after doing all of this fighting, and getting nothing. I get frustrated. When that happens, I concentrate on my other tasks. I take care of my children, do my housework, do my ASHA work, relax a little!
>
> But the women in my union won't let me leave it there. They call me, they tell me "No Anita, get up and fight."

And so she does.

"Our Union Can't Stop Us"

Not every ASHA was involved with a union—although most ASHAs agreed with the unions' goals, many felt uncomfortable with protesting, were uninterested in paying dues, or just didn't trust the leaders. One Anganwadi Worker and her husband—who were both angry over the issue of low pay and a lack of benefits—discussed this issue with us:

SVEA: Were you ever involved in the union?

ANGANWADI WORKER: I went to a meeting once, but they don't achieve anything.

HUSBAND: Those union people, they only think of themselves. They don't really do much for anybody else.

ANGANWADI WORKER: How many times do they ask women to protest every year? They make all these promises, but then they do nothing. The ASHAs went on a hunger strike, for twelve days, and one of them died.

A substantial number of ASHAs, though, *were* involved with unions. When we asked them which union they belonged to, almost none of them could name the overall leader. They named their local leaders, women that included Anita and Meena. By asking these local leaders which union they were affiliated with, we followed these threads to six different union organizations claiming to represent the ASHAs of Rajasthan.

All six of these organizations were run by men. Most were affiliated with political parties; a few were led by men who planned to run for political office. Some of these unions were large and powerful; some were anemic.

We interviewed the leaders of all six of these unions. They had a few things in common. First, they were all eloquent and compelling on the topic of minimum wage laws and ASHA pay. One union leader held forth:

> If we talk about the minimum wage, if we talk about the Labor Act, the ASHAs, the Anganwadi Workers, the Anganwadi Helpers, they haven't benefited from it. And this isn't fair. Look, they follow mothers through their pregnancies, and then they follow the child for five years to make sure they are healthy and fed. But after all that, the ASHA can't afford to provide for her own child. Because the Indian government is not caring for her, that's why these women are under a heavy burden.

Another declared: "We are fighting for them to become government employees. And until the day that they become government employees, they should get the minimum wage of eighteen thousand [rupees a month]. They should get that. But they're not even getting that. And that's what we're fighting for. We continue the fight."

Every union leader described their commitment to achieving the labor rights of ASHAs. We often got the sense during these interviews that we were listening to well-rehearsed speeches. These leaders had made these pitches many times before. This is not to say that the leaders were disingenuous; but it was very hard to discern where they personally stood on these issues.

Another commonality among all six union leaders was that they did not get along with the leaders of the *other* unions. Each claimed that *their* union was the one that truly represented ASHAs' interests.

The result was that the ASHA labor movement was fragmented. Splintered among six unions, some more popular in certain regions or among certain groups than others, there was not a unified group that could pull the ASHA voices together.

Anita commented, "The ASHAs have no leader. No place where all fifty thousand of us can come together. It would be better for the ASHAs if we were all together in one place, if we had just one union."

Anita was dissatisfied by the status quo. She tried to work around it as much as she could by encouraging ASHAs to show up to whatever protests seemed likely to bear fruit, regardless of whether she was affiliated with that union or not. "You can't stop ASHAs," she argued, "we are all together. We'll show up. Our union can't stop us. If our union's leaders tell us not to go to another protest, we'll say, 'No, actually, you should be joining us there. Why aren't you doing anything?'"

This issue—the fact that ASHAs were divided among six unions and thus did not have a unified voice—seemed to us a critical issue with their gaining enough power to enact change. But aside from a few leaders like Anita, most ASHAs were not focused on this issue. Many were not aware of it at all.

In contrast, most ASHAs' concerns about the union were focused on the issue of dues. Like Meena, ASHAs were very focused on what was being done with their truly hard earned money. Meena's concerns about Shafique using the union to line his own pockets were deep, and they were shared by many other ASHAs.

Anita shared this concern. She also used it to convince women to follow *her* rather than other union leaders.

Anita's Story III: "Something has to go into their pockets. Otherwise, why will they fight for us?"

Another union leader, Shafique, he is also taking money from women. Once he asked me to meet him, and then when I got there, he was taking 500 rupees apiece from the women in his union.

I said to him, "These are poor women! If they had 500 rupees to spare, would they need to be standing out on the street protesting?" I said, "Shafique, you are doing wrong by these women."

And then he took the money and went to Mecca for the Hajj! For a month! He was gone for a month, and I met with all of his ASHAs. I told them, "Shafique took your money. He didn't do anything for you—he took your money and went to Saudi Arabia." Then all of those women came to *our* union.

All of the union leaders, they are just looking out for themselves (*khud kī dharmśālā hai*). All their expenses, they get it from the union.

We ASHAs recently told Shiv Partap that we are going to start doing our own accounting. We're skilled enough! If we are going to give someone money, we are going to keep track of it. Who spent how much. And how much is left. So next time there is a protest, we're not going to give those leaders even one rupee.

Right? We are poor women, we are widows, we are women whose husbands have left, we are divorced women, poor women like me, where are we going to come up with money, again and again? That's why we started telling the union leaders, we can't give any more than 300 rupees a year apiece.

We tell Shiv Partap, "We collected 300 rupees from each woman. Take it, *and* then you had better tell us from that total, what you spent, and where. And how much is left. And then next time, we'll give you what you spent. But not more."

Recently we did a protest, in October. Shiv Partap didn't come, we weren't getting along. The reason was that he had told us he wanted a pension! We told him that before we were going to give him *that*, he needed to do the accounting for all of [his] previous expenditures.

He told us, "There's not a single rupee left. I spent so much out of my own pocket."

I said, "If you spent that much, then what did you spend it on? You need to tell us that."

But he wouldn't share his accounts. He didn't give us that information, and when the next protest was about to happen, he said, "It won't happen without money."

We said, "We won't give more money without any accounting," and then he didn't do anything.

He's all about money. He *dies* for money.

But look, I'm realistic. If there's no benefit at all to the union leaders, they won't do this in the first place. If the ASHA salary gets raised, then we benefit. But the union leaders don't. So *something* has to go into their pockets. Otherwise, why will they fight for us?

Take Shiv Partap. He's running a union, that's how he gets a *bhaumāt* [group of supporters], and when he shows that, the political parties might give him a ticket to run for office. He can show that he has so many followers, in all these areas of Rajasthan. It's planning for *that* future that he organizes the union in the first place. Recently, he went to [a major party] trying to get a ticket. But they didn't choose him.

Anyway, he is helping us get our work done. If we have problems, he sorts them out. One day he will get a ticket from a party. And we will vote for him.

When we are fighting for our rights, if we help him win an election, maybe he'll do even more for us.

Political Ties, Political Ambitions

Anita was right that Shafique and Shiv Partap had political aspirations. While there might be a bit of money to be made from dues, and while union leaders might be legitimately committed to promoting the rights of ASHAs (it was hard to spend much time with these ASHAs and *not* be), political ambitions were clearly a key motivator for many of the men who ran the ASHA unions. Even union leaders not formally affiliated with a political party, like Shafique, were doing what Anita described—using their union following to try to convince a party to give them a spot on the ballot.

Shafique did not just have an ASHA union—he had others as well, from Anganwadi Workers to rickshaw drivers. While he told us he had no political ambitions, we heard from other sources that he was angling for a political seat—that in fact he was open to being part of BJP or Congress, ideology mattered less than acceptance. His strategies were working: one of his family members, over the course of our project, was elected into a local political position through a major party.

These facts—that each party had its own union, and that union leaders unaffiliated with political parties were often hoping to gain such an affiliation—had two effects that worked against ASHA voice. The first was that, as mentioned earlier, these dynamics fragmented ASHAs into many different unions all competing for their participation.

But there was a deeper, more disturbing dynamic as well. The political party in power often had reasons to want ASHAs *not* to succeed in their ambitions of higher pay and job security: after all, it was their government that would have to pay for those things. So, our respondents repeatedly commented, whatever party was in power at a given time sometimes attempted to use its unions to convince ASHAs to be *silent* about their complaints. In effect, the unions could work *against* rather than for them.

In fact, this is a fairly common dynamic in Indian unions, particularly for contingent workers like ASHAs. In many cases, unions in India represent permanent, regularized workers, excluding contract labor from collective bargaining.[7] In this sense, the success of ASHAs and Anganwadi Workers in being pulled into established unions is notable, likely due to political parties' awareness that having huge numbers of rural women on their side could be useful.

Unions, though, are sophisticated political entities playing a "complicated game."[8] In some cases, unions can value close relationships with employers over the interests of their weakest members and can actively work against them; some corrupt union leaders can even be complicit in safeguarding corporate profit over worker welfare.[9]

Overall, unions in India *do* benefit the workers they represent. They can put political pressure on powerful corporations, making sure that labor laws are enforced.[10] Overall, ASHAs felt that unionizing had been generally beneficial. But the ASHAs with more experience with the unions also felt that union leaders put their own political interests ahead of the ASHAs' interests. Our observations bore this out.

"We Put the Nation First, and the Workers Second"

A leader of yet another union discussed this issue at length. He pointed at the BJP and Congress-affiliated unions as deeply problematic. Each of them advocated strongly for ASHAs when they were not in control in the government, he observed. But the party that *was* controlling the government—the same government that was the employer of the ASHAs—was a different story.

> [The party in power] will tell the people in their unions: *do not go on strike.*
>
> The union leaders are mostly all after political tickets. Shafique will get a ticket. Shiv Partap wants one. . . . I'll never take a ticket, although the BJP likes me, and so does Congress. Because if I were to also be a politician, I wouldn't reach the goals for ASHAs that I am fighting for.

Whether or not it is true that this respondent would turn down a party position if it were offered him, his analysis lines up with ours, and with what union leaders affiliated with the ruling party themselves said in interviews. A union leader affiliated with the party in power explained that he discouraged the ASHAs in his union from going on strike, although they did demonstrate:

> We don't strike. That's not our method. Because we're such a large union, and the second thing is, the other unions don't have the reach ours do.
>
> We have so much power that the government has to listen to us. Those who

strike, they're hurting the country. . . . We work for the benefit of our nation. We put the nation first, and the workers, second.

These dynamics—that the unions were closely affiliated with the very political parties who were running the government and, by extension, the ASHA program, put the male union leaders in a complex place. ASHAs who had the most experience with the unions, like Anita, were well aware of this.

Anita's Story, IV: "We ASHAs Pressure Them from One Side, but Their Parties Pressure Them from the Other"

I say to Shiv Partap, "Your government is in power. Why aren't you doing anything for us?"

But here's what happens. We ASHAs pressure the union leaders from one side, but their parties pressure them from the other. And then they turn on us. They say to us, "You're part of our party, it's disrespectful to protest."

When the opposition party was in power, Shiv Partap put on great protests. He would say openly, "We will jam the road." But when his party came into power, he quieted his protests.

They tell us one thing, but then when they meet with the ministers they're doing something else.

And then they give us just enough to dismiss our concerns. Here's how they think: "Ten, twenty rupees, give it to them, they'll be quiet. What do poor women need? We'll toss them a crumb and they'll be quiet." That's how it goes.

"If the ASHAs Stop Working, It Will Destroy the Government"

On the day we sat in Shiv Partap's office, he weaved a narrative with himself as the protagonist: a passionate advocate for ASHA and Anganwadi rights, navigating the frustrating lack of motion on the part of government bureaucrats. He pointed out that *shiskha karmis*, village-level female education workers who had also previously been categorized as volunteers, had been given permanent positions. He also pointed out that servants in households were also now mandated to get minimum wage. He was trying, he said, to get the government to extend the same logic to ASHAs and Anganwadi Workers: "But there's only so much we can do. We can be with them, we can help with their demands, but if the Rajasthani government doesn't agree, then what can we do?"

All of this was met with enthusiastic agreement and discussion by the other men in the room—affirming Shiv Partap's ideas and actions. One told Shiv Partap, "You should run for the legislative assembly!"

Shiv Partap at first demurred, pointing to the sizable salary and pension he enjoyed in his current government job. "But," he added, "if someone from the party comes to me, I might run."

It was then that the conversation in the room took a revealing turn. Everyone in the room agreed that if the ruling party didn't make ASHA and Anganwadi Workers permanent, it could ultimately damage them. The discussion continued from there:

> MAN 1: There are so many ASHAs, and they really know the people in the field—if they were to really stop working it would destroy the government!
>
> MAN 2: Don't give that idea to the opposition!
>
> MAN 1: There are 150,000 of them [in Rajasthan], and these are women that know every house. They potentially have a lot of power. They have been following every child since before the children were born, they get those children vaccinated, they follow them until they are five years old.
>
> MAN 3, LAUGHING NERVOUSLY: You will destroy us if you give them that idea!
>
> SHIV PARTAP: It's not an idle idea. I'm telling you, I'm the person who is meeting with these women. Why do you not realize this? This is what will happen if you don't do something for them.

The men in the room were arguing not to empower ASHAs, but to *keep* them from recognizing their political power. The fear of an ASHA uprising in the room was real—it would "destroy the government." Shiv Partap tread an interesting line in his response—that "doing something" for ASHAs was necessary in order to avoid the threat of social unrest.

These same ideas had in fact already occurred to ASHAs themselves. Over time, the ASHA leaders involved with these unions became increasingly aware that they might have to defy union leaders to reach their goals—that going on strike might be a more effective way of drawing attention to their needs than following the directives of union leaders to protest in more quiet ways. Anita commented:

Without us, they'll never control measles, they'll never control rubella. We ASHAs have all the information, nobody else knows the kids. The ANM doesn't know this information. They might have some records, but they can't do much with that. We're in touch with the people.

Yes, children's lives are in the balance. We told them, we only make Rs 2,500, we can't make it all work. Some of us are divorced, we have to do everything with just Rs 2,500 a month. We can't even feed our own children. If other kids are harmed because we don't work, well, let it happen, we have our own children too!

Anita was not alone in these musings. Another ASHA union leader we spoke to, her words echoing those of the men in the government office, explained passionately, "If the ASHAs were to stop working it would destroy the government!"

Anita's Story, V: "We Will Be Our Own Leaders"

So I am thinking, how long will we chase after these leaders? We should make our own union, standing on our own legs. And ASHAs, we will fight, ourselves.

I have been calling other ASHAs who have been union leaders. There are three of us who know all the ASHAs of Rajasthan. We have the contacts. We have the knowledge. We have met with these women. We have called them.

Years ago I didn't have the knowledge of how to lead a union, but I have learned. We've watched Shiv Partap, we've watched the other leaders, and we women have learned. We're ready to shoot for the moon, we ASHAs.

We won't bring any other leaders. We will be our own leaders. We will be ASHAs. We will be powerful. We won't bring any leaders with us. We will do it all ourselves.

At home, we ASHAs may not be anything. But we are learning about our own power outside. We are ready to bring back the moon and stars.

CHAPTER 6

Our Union Can't Stop Us

Leaving the Unions Behind

We had heard a lot about Seema before we met her. We heard things like: Seema wasn't going to follow the directions of male union leaders. Seema had some risky tactics. Seema might make herself the ASHAs' new leader.

Seema's house was in a dilapidated section of the Old City of Jaipur. The alleyways in this part of town were too narrow for a car to navigate, so we got out of our Uber and walked through the narrow paths to Seema's house.

We met in her small cement room off of a small shared courtyard. Seema lived in this room with her two children; she shared a kitchen, another small room next door, with her neighbor. Seema's home was tiny, her existence constrained. But her personality and her dreams were huge.

Seema had called two of her co-conspirators, Ruchita and Jeevika, to talk with us as well. The five of us sat in the small, dark room. As we listened to the stories of these extraordinary women, our respect for them grew.

"If We Don't Raise Our Voices, Nobody Will Ever Give Us Anything"

"Our goal is this," Seema explained. "If the government isn't going to listen, we'll protest. It's simple."

And, she added, the three of them had decided that it was time for more militant methods—that peaceful protesting was not achieving enough: "If a baby doesn't cry, the mother won't feed it! If we don't raise our voices, nobody will ever give us anything. If we don't say anything, if we don't do anything, will the government give us anything?"

Tired of what they saw as the ineffective methods of the established unions, Seema, Ruchita and Jeevika had decided to take action on their own. First, they held a strike for sixteen days—just the three of them—outside state offices in Jaipur.

Then, they leapt in front of the Chief Minister's car. "We made a plan, we will stop their car, so that at least they will listen," Jeevika explained.

But, the Chief Minister didn't listen. Instead, the Minister called the police to intervene. For this, Seema, Ruchita and Jeevika were put on probation for six months and suspended from ASHA work for three months.

Another time, when police tried to block buses full of ASHAs from gathering at a protest site, the three of them took action. "We had set up a barricade, we were stopping traffic," Seema remembered. "From one side, Ruchita was stopping cars, from the other side, me."

This didn't last long—the police swiftly arrested Seema. When the other ASHAs continued to try to stop traffic, the police took additional action. "You know those jail vehicles?" Ruchita asked. "They just packed them full of ASHAs and carted us off." Seema, Ruchita, and Jeevika were briefly jailed. But, because they had been on a hunger strike for a week, they ultimately were delivered to the hospital and were sent home with another three-month work suspension.

This three-month work suspension did not succeed in getting Seema, Ruchita, and Jeevika to stop their agitating. Rather, desperate to get their work back, they explained to us that they had no choice but to take additional steps.

RUCHITA: We tried to meet with the ICDS director [state officer responsible for Anganwadi Centers] in her office. But she wouldn't give us a meeting. One day as she was showing up to work in her car, we stopped her car, to say, listen to us. She said, "Don't stop the car!" and she cursed us out.
JEEVIKA: She cursed my mother!
RUCHITA: And she lifted up her hand and told us she was going to slap us.
JEEVIKA: Oh, then it was ON. We were going to fight. I grabbed onto a nearby gate, so nobody could pull me away from the car, and we started exchanging curses. Well, she called the police. And they arrested us and took us to the police station. And *this* time, they had filed an FIR against us.

An FIR (First Information Report) is the first step in a criminal prosecution. But the threat of legal action did not make these women back down.

Instead, they fought back: Seema, Ruchita, and Jeevika themselves filed an FIR against the ICDS director. This tactic worked, they said: they got their jobs back in exchange for stopping legal action.

"Who Will Care for Us? Nobody Will Care."

What was striking about the actions of these women—and very different from the tactics of the established unions connected to political parties—was their take-no-prisoners approach. Rather than follow the directions of a male, politically connected union leader, Seema and her friends were attempting to take matters into their own hands. They did so because they had little to lose: Seema was raising her children on her own, existing on the very ragged edge of total poverty. And, they explained, they felt neglected by the systems that employed them.

> RUCHITA: Nobody cares for us. If we get swine flu while doing the survey of flu patients, then what medical care will we get? Who will care for us? Nobody will care.
>
> JEEVIKA: In 2016, during a polio campaign, I wasn't feeling well. I told my supervisor, "Sir, I can't do the polio campaign. My health is really bad." They told me, "Bring a written order from a higher level officer, if you want to get out of the work."
>
> That officer wouldn't give me a written order, so I ran here, I ran there, I did the polio campaign one day, and on the second day while I was on the road, I got really sick. They took me to the hospital, put me in the ICU [Intensive Care Unit]. I got three bottles of blood. But look, the people at the hospital, my supervisors in the office, not one of them called me, not one asked: What happened to the ASHA? Is she okay?
>
> Whose responsibility is that? When we are sick, our supervisors put pressure on us. And when we end up in the hospital, they can't even be bothered to pick up the phone. Why do they treat us like that?

Seema, Ruchita, and Jeevika had decided that a more militant approach was likely to be the most effective. In this, their approach differed sharply from that of Meena and Anita. What all of these women had in common, though, was a growing feeling that they would need to move beyond the existing union structures if they were really to make the most of the potential power of Rajasthan's extensive network of ASHAs.

Three Women, Three Approaches, Three Common Frustrations

Seema had different tactics from Anita, and a completely different orientation from Meena. But all three women, despite their very different personalities and philosophies, shared some common frustrations.

Meena was under increasing pressure from other ASHAs to show results for the union dues she had collected on behalf of her union leader, Shafique. Of the forty or so ASHAs she worked with on a regular basis, all but five had given her Rs 1,500 (more than $20) apiece to contribute to union activities—a large amount of money for many of these women. And, she had also collected dues from ASHAs in the neighboring areas. It was becoming a problem for her, she explained:

> There has been no benefit. Shafique told us, it will take time. It will take six months, a year, he said, and then you'll see the result of my legal action. Believing that, we thought, well, we can spare Rs 1,500. We all gave him the money. Those of us who are leaders, *we* collected the money from everyone.
>
> But, our salary has not changed. A few of the women understand, the rest don't understand. They gave money; they're angry with Shafique.

Meena was as committed as ever to working toward a permanent, well-paid position for ASHAs. But, she was nearing the end of her patience with the union structures:

> Shafique just wants the parties to pick him for a ticket, for the legislative assembly. I'm telling you. Whenever there's a chance for a photo op or a TV recording, he's there, speaking. If not, he doesn't do anything. He wants to show that yes, I'm here, I have all these followers. I'm telling you the truth, he's just using ASHAs for his own benefit.
>
> When the discussions about the budget were happening, he wasn't even in the country! And after that, we didn't hear anything from him. Then how can we believe he's fighting for us? He's just fighting for himself. That's why none of us are happy with Shafique these days.

Meena was angry: her time, her effort, and her legitimacy were all on the line. She feared that her efforts were evaporating, serving only to support Shafique's political candidacy, and not doing much for ASHAs. She wanted things to change.

Anita had also reached the point of frustration—for similar reasons, but with a different union leader. Because Anganwadi Workers' pay had recently been raised, but ASHAs' had not, she was increasingly feeling like ASHAs were not a priority.

"When it comes to representing the ASHAs," she said, "they just collect money from us, and that's all. They tell us, 'I will do this for you, that for you,' but they don't. . . . So that's why ASHAs are irritated. But still, some foolish ASHAs continue to follow Shiv Partap. More aggressive ASHAs like me, we are not joining with him any more."

Seema, Ruchita, and Jeevika had already decided to go out on their own. So far it had not borne fruit: they had been arrested and suspended, but unlike Shafique and Shiv Partap, who were usually able to get a few minutes with a government official on the day a strike took place, they had yet to have a conversation with anyone in power.

The Protest that Flopped

A few weeks after we visited Seema at home, Meena, Anita, and Seema all attended the same protest. We found them all, with several hundred other ASHAs, massed in an unlikely venue: a closed gas station. There was no tent and no microphone; women milled around the defunct petrol pumps. Construction work was going on in the adjacent lot, so even when someone tried to give a speech, it was almost impossible to hear them. The problem was with the permission to congregate: "They cancelled it," Meena explained. "The authorities told us last night that our request to assemble in the original place was denied. That nobody would be allowed to be there." Gathering at the abandoned gas station had been a last minute decision; the police had said that since ASHAs were arriving from all over Rajasthan, they would be allowed to meet there.

This protest was disappointing for everyone: a smaller turnout than anyone had hoped, and a distinctly uninspiring venue. Many women had paid for bus and train tickets from distant parts of Rajasthan, and this was not the outcome they had imagined. Meena commented:

Everybody knew about it! It was even in the newspaper. It was on the news. They said it would be a very big strike. But there weren't that many people. Everyone was without hope. And everyone has been fragmented into different unions. Shafique has one, Seema has another. There's another from another area of Rajasthan, so people have been distributed across all these different unions. If everyone was together, if all the ASHAs were together, then you would see a result!

The frustration of the ASHAs with the disappointing protest—a "flop," some commented—turned into frustration with union leaders, particularly with Shafique, who showed up at the protest but, many women commented, was only active in front of the TV cameras.

As they always did when holding protests, some union leaders (in this case Meena and Seema) went with a written list of their demands to the government health department offices. Politically connected union leaders could usually get a meeting of at least a few minutes. But Meena couldn't get past the guards, who told them the minister wasn't there and took the paper with promises they would pass it on. Meena was not hopeful, and neither was Seema or Ruchita.

The frustrated energy in the air was palpable: it was a mix of aggression and exhaustion among the ASHAs. There were a few reporters in attendance, and the ASHAs in front of the TV cameras were doing their best to demonstrate their power. "An ASHA can tell everyone whether the government's policies are good or bad," one ASHA said into the camera, "and the ASHA can *also* tell them not to vote for the BJP government." Amid this disappointing showing, she was pushing hard to illuminate the potential political power of a unified bloc of ASHAs.

But the ASHAs were *not* unified—or not yet. "All of the ASHAs will have to work together," Meena commented: "Otherwise, it doesn't matter what you do, nothing will happen. When all the ASHAs are together, something can happen. . . . Seema was saying the same thing—bring all the unions together."

Seema was ready and waiting to take advantage of this situation, particularly women's mounting impatience with Shafique. She was recruiting women who had been supporting Shafique to join *her* union instead. It was working: even Meena, who was generally skeptical of Seema's more extreme tactics, was ready to leave Shafique behind and join her.

Part of Seema's strategy was to position herself as more militant and more active than Shafique. She would protest with or without permission, she told us, commenting that she told the police, "All you can do is bring me to jail. And I've already been there." She added: "Shafique said, 'we'll stay within the boundaries of the law.' But I don't think staying within the boundaries of the law will get anything done."

Seema Gives Up

After this protest, the two of us, Surendra and Svea, talked. We had hope: we thought there was potential for the creation of an independent ASHA union, by and for ASHAs, the kind of union that Meena, Anita, and Seema all hoped for. And for a while, there was energy. The women created a WhatsApp group for Rajasthan's ASHAs. It grew beyond the limits of people allowed in a single group, and it grew to five WhatsApp groups: more than a thousand women, a strong start.

But when we interviewed Seema nine months later, she had completely given up. It was all going nowhere, she said. It didn't matter what they tried—nobody would listen. Perhaps she would start an NGO (Non-Governmental Organization), she mused. There was money in that.

Seema's friend Ruchita was still trying a little. She was still angry about what she saw as lack of respect and prioritization for ASHAs. But she was frustrated.

"Nothing is coming of any of it," she told us. "Nothing at all is happening. These days, I'm not protesting at all. The ASHAs from other areas are doing this, but I'm not leading it. . . . There's no point."

The energy of these women was over, the momentum gone. Meena was also starting to move on. But Anita was still trying to bring together the ASHAs of Rajasthan on her own. One morning, we went to a protest Anita had organized in Jaipur. Anita's protest was the first we had heard of organized by ASHAs, with no politically affiliated union leaders behind the scenes.

"You Say You Want Permission, But Nobody Will Give Us Permission"

When we arrived in the area of Jaipur where Anita's protest was supposed to be, we found nothing: it seemed to be an ordinary day, with the usual traffic. After a lot of driving around, we finally found the protest: it was held on an unused side road, out of the way, completely invisible from the main streets.

This was, to say the least, not a high visibility spot for a protest. Once again, the ASHAs had been denied the necessary permissions, and had been given this spot to congregate.

The police were there; they had barricaded both ends of the road where the women were. They asked the two of us whether we were journalists; we explained that we were anthropologists, writing a book about the ASHA program, and they nodded and let us in. They explained to us, conversationally, that the women didn't have permission to congregate. But they were allowing them to stay, for the time being.

A large number of police, many of them women, sat in the shade under some tents they had erected; the protestors outnumbered the police, but not by much. Vendors had set up shop along the periphery, selling snacks and ice cream. The police had brought in a water truck and a portable toilet station. It was all very orderly, and all completely hidden from the main road.

Around noon, when we arrived, there were a couple hundred ASHAs there. Many wore the light blue government-issue ASHA saris. The sun was beating down, and they gathered in clumps on the pavement under umbrellas to shade them from the brutal heat.

Many of these women were from a remote city in Rajasthan, many hours from Jaipur. They had spent last night on an overnight train, and then they'd been out in the blazing sun on the pavement all day. The temperature was at least 40 degrees Celsius (more than 100 degrees Fahrenheit), and it was definitely hotter than that on the pavement. Most had not slept much the night before, and many were a little bleary.

This protest was part of a series of activities these women had been conducting for several weeks, when they had begun a work stoppage in their districts. They did this during the dates scheduled for a measles vaccination campaign, an activity that relies heavily on ASHAs for its implementation.

When that, along with visits to the district magistrate in their area, had failed to show results, they tried bringing their case to other government ministers. Now, they were trying to draw the attention of high-level officials in Jaipur to their cause. Their demand was almost heartbreakingly small—they were asking for a raise of Rs 500 (less than $10) per month. This seemed to us like a lot to go through to ask for such a small raise.

That morning, the leaders of the strike—Anita and a few others—had left the hidden strike area and gone to the state government buildings in hopes of getting a meeting. So everyone behind in the protest area was just waiting. The two of us attracted some attention as we arrived, and a group clustered around to talk to us—they'd come so far and had prepared their speeches, and there were few available audiences to hear them. They had come all this way to plead their case, rehearsing their talking points on the way, only to find nobody to listen. So they told *us* what they wanted government officials to hear:

> We get all the calls. When there's dengue, the ASHA is there. When there's malaria, the ASHA is there. When there's swine flu, the ASHA is there.
>
> ———
>
> The ASHAs do all the nurse's work. The nurse doesn't have the first idea of what is going on in which house. But she gets Rs. 40,000, and we get Rs. 2,500.
>
> ———
>
> If we are not doing our work well, we get in trouble for our mistakes. But we really do our work properly. Then why don't they pay us properly?
>
> ———
>
> The government says, "*betī bachāo, betī paḍhāo*" (save your daughter, educate your daughter), but at 2,500 rupees a month, how can we possibly educate our daughters?
>
> ———
>
> We're the only workers the government doesn't seem to be able to find space for in their budgets.

A plainclothes police officer was getting similar speeches from the assembled women; he listened sympathetically and walked around the crowd in a friendly way. The uniformed police officers primarily sat to the side in the shade of their tents.

Some of the police officers were explaining to the frustrated ASHAs how to get actual permission to congregate. "To get permission," one explained, "you need to go through the Chief Minister's office. Then there would be a record of your request. Then everything would be working properly. You need to follow the system!"

The women argued that they did send an email requesting permission, but no response came. The police officer said it couldn't be done by email. One woman, frustrated, cried out, "You say you want permission, but nobody will give us permission. So we did the protest without permission."

Several women commented that this seemed to be a coordinated government strategy. When they requested permission through the proper channels, it was denied. And when they assembled without a permit, they were told that their protest wasn't legitimate. They were allowed to assemble—the police were extraordinarily skilled at avoiding confrontation—but they were reminded that they didn't have the right to be there.

Regardless of whether obtaining permission would have been "easy" for ASHAs, as the police officer claimed, what was clear was that without a politically connected and bureaucratically savvy leader—someone like Shiv Partap—holding a high profile event was extraordinarily difficult. The ASHAs, working alone without powerful political backing, were easy to sideline.

A Slow Defeat

As the day progressed and everyone grew exhausted from standing in the heat, we sat on the pavement with a group of women. They all scooted closer together to make room for us on the old plastic banner they had spread on the pavement to sit on. A couple ASHAs were lying down on the edges of the banner, under the shade of umbrellas. We asked the women if they thought anything will come of this today, of their coming all the way here. "Who knows?" they said. They didn't seem that hopeful.

One woman, skeletally thin, was supporting her family through ASHA work, and she stopped to wipe away tears as she talked about her frustrations with her low pay. The group discussed the fact that Anganwadi Workers had recently gotten a pay raise, while ASHAs had not. It was tearing them apart, the group commented. One of the more voluble women in the group opined sardonically, "They took a lesson from the British: divide and rule."

Suddenly the beating sun was replaced by a downpour. Some clusters of women on the pavement doubled down under their umbrellas, holding them close together in an attempt to keep out the deluge. Others scattered.

When the storm passed, the relentless sun came out again. It was exhausting, to sit on the pavement battered by the weather.

The afternoon wore on, slowly. Anita and four other women had left in the morning to plead their case with the government officials in charge of the ASHA program; they were still waiting to see someone, they told us (and others) by text message. The crowd was tired and seemed to be dwindling a little.

In the end, Anita waited all day in the Assembly building and only met an administrative assistant—the entire day was basically a waste. She and the women with her weren't given access to any political leaders.

Around 4:30, Anita and her fellow leaders returned. They were frustrated, near tears. They lead the tired group in some chants, and then they chatted with us, sad and dejected. "What should we do, Surendra?" one asked.

There was another downpour; we huddled together under umbrellas. When it cleared, we talked for a bit, and then the police began to clear us out. They did a sweep of the space, male and female officers in brown uniforms walking slowly in a semicircle to push the assembled ASHAs out onto the main road.

There was no confrontation; the police didn't have to say anything. The ASHAs walked in front of the police, leaving. The mood was one of dejection. Some women said they would go back to their own cities and do hunger strikes.

In the morning, the women had been fired up. But making their leaders wait in the government offices was an effective method of tiring out a group of ASHAs already exhausted from an overnight train ride. The ASHAs' energy had been efficiently managed, their modest demands for a 500 rupee raise tamped down.

Later, we talked to Anita about the protest. She commented that it was hard to protest in Jaipur because Jaipur's ASHAs, having had negative repercussions from protesting in the past, were now reluctant to attend protests: "The ASHAs of Jaipur city, they won't protest. Partly because all of the protests happen here, and they are tired. They say, 'The women from out of town will just leave. But after the protest, we'll get harassed by our officers.' So Jaipur's ASHAs, they won't protest. Not even one. The ones from the villages, they come. But the ASHAs from the cities, they don't show up."

Still, Anita hadn't given up hope. "All of the ASHAs are ready," she said, "to create a unified front."

Nonetheless, the fact remained that AHSA-led organizing was not going far. Anita and Seema and Meena were all deeply limited by the fact that they did not have political connections of any kind. Working on their own, they were unable to make inroads into power structures. They were easy to marginalize, to literally push to the side in abandoned petrol pumps and abandoned lots. The fundamental lack of power of ASHA organizers, combined with the enormous political savvy of Rajasthani government and political institutions, made it extremely difficult for them to make any progress on their own. The ASHAs were ready to fight. But powerful actors were also ready to shut them down. And so intelligent, charismatic, and committed women like Anita experienced a series of defeats.

Protests after COVID

After that conversation with Anita, the COVID pandemic hit. So it was a while before we had a chance to follow up again about the trajectory of the unions.

In 2022, India's ASHAs won the WHO Director General's Global Health Leaders Award for their work during COVID. This was, of course, well deserved. The video released by WHO commemorating this called the ASHAs "a million champions of health and hope." It also called them "volunteers."

But what was particularly interesting about the discourse around this award was that, for the first time we had seen on a broad scale, ASHAs were hailed not just as selfless champions but as workers deserving of a living wage. An article published in the South-East Asian wing of the *Lancet* commented that award "should be considered an opportunity for the global health community and policy makers to reflect on the relative power and agency of ASHAs in the hierarchical and power laden health systems in India."[1] An article about the award in the Indian newspaper *The Hindu* highlighted ASHA protests, and their demands for a living wage and regular work.[2] And several international unions that we had never run across in Rajasthan argued passionately on Twitter that this award was a reason to support ASHA unionization. So it seemed to us, from our quarantine seats in front of our respective computers in Baltimore and Jaipur, as if things might be changing.

But when we talked with the ASHAs we knew after the pandemic had passed, the online energy had not tricked down to Gurha Sajjanpura. Bharti said she hadn't heard of a strike since 2019—"we were thinking about striking during COVID, but we did nothing," she commented.

Kavita had heard of some more recent protests, but hadn't participated. She didn't think there was a point. "I don't think there's any way the government will listen to us," she said. "The government is not going to do anything."

"We Were Working During Corona, So Why Would We Be Scared Now?"

There was one ASHA, Priya, who had always been involved in unions, but who had become more deeply involved after COVID. The intense work and risk that ASHAs had taken on in the pandemic had pushed her toward greater involvement.

Priya went to protests that were organized by another ASHA. That leader was using tactics that reminded us of Seema. But the outcome was familiar too.

Priya told us about it:

That leader showed a lot of courage. She came all the way from rural Rajasthan, and the police didn't let us have a place to protest. They said we didn't have permission. So that ASHA said to the police, "Get rid of us! Do whatever you want to do!"

We did this protest during COVID, in the cold months. People said to us, you'll get Corona. So many ASHAs were all in the same place. But we were working during Corona, so why would we be scared now?

And then the police kept telling us: If you stand here in the cold and the rain, you'll get sick. The police also said to us, it's not as if you are wrong in your demands, but the government is not going to listen to you. Some of the police prayed for us, "Hey Bhagavan, tell the government to listen to the ASHAs."

At some point we got an appointment with the Chief Minister. But they went to Delhi, instead of meeting with us. When we came back from the government office, the police asked us how it went. "They didn't listen to us," we told them. "No one ever listens to us."

Some minister from the Secretariat, he gave us some blankets. It was raining. We were huddled under a tree. We slept on the cold footpath. In seventeen years of working, that was the hardest thing I've done. But I got used to sleeping on the footpath. I got used to eating, there, on the road.

In the end, the police filed a case against us. I was crying. It was so sad, they didn't stand with us. God stayed with us, we didn't get sick. We scolded the police, when they took us to jail.

Now, the ASHAs have also given up hope. Because our leader was fired from her job as an AHSA. Fired for standing up for us. Everything is a waste.

All of us, we are tired.

We women are tired of being afraid.

CONCLUSION

Toward Truly Supported Community Health Workers

At the beginning of this book, we posed the questions: How does ASHA work shift gender relations within the family? How and when do ASHAs push back against power structures in the family, and in the health system, and what happens when they do? Are unions a way of shifting these power dynamics?

The shifts in ASHAs' family structures were profound. They were a result of senior family members, particularly mothers- and fathers-in-law, supporting ASHAs' mobility in the hopes that this support would ultimately lead to their daughters-in-law getting permanent government positions. The ASHAs themselves did not push very hard for these changes; they happened because there was the promise of good employment sometime in the future.

As ASHAs' families endeavored to support them in their work, the ASHAs' worlds expanded: Anju got a motor scooter. Meena started guiding her family when traveling to faraway cities for medical care. And Meena and Anita became leaders, gathering women together across the state of Rajasthan. This kind of public, mobile work was worlds away from where these women had started out, as daughters-in-law who were scared to leave the house.

Because ASHA work was honorable, it allowed women to stretch some of the usual bonds of respectability, traveling not only to local health centers, but to cities. While senior family members still ultimately made decisions about whether these women would do the work at all, the work expanded women's worlds in deeply meaningful ways.

Power structures within the health system were slower to bend. If ASHAs' families quickly recognized their promise and their capabilities, it felt to many ASHAs as if the health system was slower in this recognition, despite the important work they did. When ASHAs began to demand labor rights, they found their progress limited. They often found themselves entangled in power structures they could not control, and in some cases had trouble comprehending.

The established unions in Rajasthan, those affiliated with political parties, gave ASHAs an important voice. They gave them a conduit to presenting their demands to people in power. They likely played some important role in the series of raises ASHAs have received over the years. But many union leaders could at times put their own interests ahead of ASHAs' interests.

And ASHAs' attempts to move out on their own—lead by women of strong will and shimmering intellect—hit hard boundaries. Without high-level political connections, the ASHAs' attempts at collective action were easy for the state to defuse and shut down. Progress was hard to come by.

Delivered by Women, Led by Men

The controversies about what CHWs should be have existed as long as there have been formal CHWs. Should they be community-based health activists? Or should they be health system extenders, providing services? And what happens in practice: are they exploited or empowered?

Understanding CHWs' stories helps complicate these dichotomies. ASHAs are lackeys, harshly criticized when they fail to report data in the proper format, *and* they are liberators, working together for labor rights. They are of and for the health system, focusing on the limited tasks—mostly centered around maternal and child health—for which they get monetary incentives. And, simultaneously, they are of and for the people, laboring to help their neighbors file the paperwork that will allow them to get entitlements from the state.

The ASHAs we talked to did not have much of an opinion on the lackey-or-liberator question. It was clear enough to them in their day-to-day work that they were employees of the health system, government staff. Their demand was simply that they be *treated* with the respect and recognition of employees. They wanted a living wage, basic benefits, a small retirement pension. Many ASHAs felt—and we agree—that it was *these* things: a wage, benefits, recognition and respect within their workplaces, that would really empower them.

Yet their attempts to change these structures were profoundly limited by the same dynamics that had created them in the first place. The World Health Organization has pointed out that global health structures are "delivered by women, led by men."[1] Although there were some influential women in leadership roles in the Indian health system, this was largely true of the ASHA program. And it was also true of the unions the ASHAs joined in their attempts to change the system.

When we started this work, we were interested in how unions might function as a powerful avenue for ASHAs to gain labor rights. But unionization is unfortunately not as straightforward a way forward as we had hoped when we began this research. Naively, we imagined that unions could be a powerful way for workers to gain voice. At times they were helpful; but for the most part gendered and classed structures kept ASHAs from gaining much power within unions, who were for the most part serving the interests of powerful men. When ASHAs tried to go out on their own, those same gendered and classed structures kept them from making much headway; without political connections, they couldn't gain access to any of the officials who could take action on wages or working conditions. And the health system itself made union leadership a risky proposition for ASHAs, who could be suspended for being too vocal.[2]

Changes in Family Structures

But change *was* happening. Rural Indian households are often constructed as bastions of traditionalism, in contrast to the modernity represented by phenomena like women's education and employment.[3] But because of the opportunities created for rural women by the ASHA and Anganwadi programs, it was in the Rajasthani family where shifts in gendered roles were in fact taking place.

Women's employment in rural Rajasthan is embedded in families in profound ways. The extent of this embeddedness is frequently not considered in programs aiming to provide income opportunities for rural women in India.[4] Yet understanding ASHAs' labor requires going beyond only thinking of work as something that happens outside the home.

In this context, the work many ASHAs did at "home" was far more economically productive for the family than the work they did at "work." Having a family member work as an ASHA could be a net economic loss for families with productive agricultural operations. Putting a woman in an ASHA position was a decision made by older family members. It was a family gamble, an income diversification strategy based on the hope that the ASHA position would eventually become a permanent job.

It was striking to us how much family structures changed as a result of women's ASHA work. They were given mobility, a partial reprieve from some of their work within the home, control over a bit of money. These shifts were not total—young married women were still the least powerful actors within Rajasthani family structures—but they were nonetheless very meaningful for the ASHAs we knew. If these shifts happened as a result of the promise of potentially someday getting a permanent government position, we think that *actually* having a permanent government position could lead to quite significant shifts in family power for young rural women in places like Rajasthan.

Of course, if ASHA jobs were to become permanent, with a living wage and benefits, the job would suddenly become even more attractive to women from a given village's most powerful families. This would shift who was able to become an ASHA—it might become out of reach of some less privileged families. Still, we think way forward here is *more* opportunity for young, educated, ambitious rural women to have living wage jobs, not less opportunity.

Managing Data

There are also some broader theoretical lessons from the experiences of the ASHAs we know. A first set of theoretical points relates to paperwork. ASHAs filled out multiple and proliferating registers and apps, reflective of demands for data and accountability from many different health programs. These data collection systems had a range of impacts, most of them not intended by the people who designed them.

In health systems across the world, data collection and management can eclipse patient care.[5] There are many examples in the anthropological literature of data collection that exemplifies technocratic, top-down global health work that is divorced from local needs.[6] Some of the voluminous bureaucratic work that the ASHAs in Rajasthan do is obviously a poor use of their time, designed to serve bureaucrats rather than community members. Arima Mishra is right when she argues that this data system reflects the Indian health system's "privileging of statistical over experiential knowledge and its reliance on top-down channels of communication."[7]

But the story also has more layers. ASHAs found pragmatic ways to deal with the bureaucratic, top-down data collection system. They estimated numbers in cases where they knew that the issue was not a critical one, and where it clearly didn't matter for patient care. The result was that the story of data collection was more complex than simply a top-down system managing ASHAs through data collection. ASHAs also managed the data system. As many anthropologists have pointed out, actors in local health systems shape data in ways that make sense given the pressures they are under; the result is that data is often less than a clear window onto local realities.[8]

Yet there was another dimension to the data collection and remuneration system, one less explored in the anthropological literature. Some of the work that this very data system pushed ASHAs to do—getting people the bank accounts and paperwork they need to access government benefits—had real, transformative potential.

Paperwork as Care Work

In the book *Red Tape,* Akhil Gupta famously argued, based in part on work with Anganwadi Workers, that bureaucratic structures put in place by the Indian government were part of what kept poverty entrenched. It was tough, he showed, for poor people to access their entitlements.[9]

Rajasthan's ASHAs were intimately familiar with this issue. Strikingly—and extremely unusually for Indian government staff—they were actively involved in solving this problem, in giving the most marginalized access to their entitlements. They advised women on filling out forms—and in many cases, they filled out forms *for* them. They advised on how to open bank accounts. They ferried paperwork from women's houses to the health center. They kept track of what had been filed and not been filed. In the process, they helped the most marginalized women in Gurha Sajjanpura access large cash entitlements that improved their lives.

In doing so, they made a real, meaningful difference in the lives of the women they served. It was not the work that the activists who framed the ASHA program envisioned. Nor was it even the activism work outlined for them in the national level training modules—as most of that material never made it into trainings in practice. The ASHAs we knew did not, as these unused training materials hoped they would, band together to stop violence against women. They did not organize for environmental justice. They did not bring women's rights issues to the *gram panchayat.*

But, by helping women access their entitlements day in and day out, Rajasthan's ASHAs did something perhaps even more profound. They helped families living close to the edge access desperately needed cash to feed, clothe, and care for their daughters. They ironed out bureaucratic obstacles to immunization, and to school enrollment for girls.

They did not do this because they were selfless; they did it because they were incentivized to do it. If a woman's paperwork was not complete, the ASHA herself could not get *her* incentives. This was a perhaps unanticipated positive consequence of the incentive-based remuneration system. We agree with many people we spoke to that perhaps giving an ASHA a wage unconnected to specific tasks would allow her to have a greater focus on the determinants of health. And, as ASHAs themselves have compellingly argued, there are important labor rights reasons to push for a reliable salary. But, the incentive based payment structure had one large positive outcome: It pushed ASHAs to help women for whom bureaucratic structures were opaque and frightening navigate those structures, and access the health-enhancing cash that was waiting for them.

Going back to Akhil Gupta's argument in *Red Tape,* if onerous bureaucratic requirements are a large part of what keeps people in India in poverty, then the work that ASHAs are doing ferrying paperwork around is potentially the most crucially important part of their jobs. It is in many ways the embodiment of one of the key roles long envisioned for CHWs: helping people navigate confusing or alien bureaucratic and health structures.

In the anthropological literature, paperwork is often seen as opposed to or a distraction from care.[10] And at times it was for the ASHAs we knew. But filling out paperwork was also an extraordinarily important way that ASHAs *provided* care. We watched as ASHAs worked very hard to ferry paperwork to and from banks, health centers, photocopy shops, and people's homes. They got the most marginalized families access to cash benefits. Meena made sure that the family whose story opens this book got a modest but steady stream of cash from the government to support their daughter. A woman without a roof, living in a cart with some blankets, got a large cash payment from the government thanks to Anju. For these families, living in enormous poverty and scarcity, without the resources to access these government entitlements on their own, these acts of care were profound.

Embracing Complexity

Another theoretical observation is the need for great care and specificity when discussing the effects of "the state." The "Indian state" is a complex and multifaceted entity, and anthropological analyses of its workings should understand what is going on on the inside as well as on the outside. In the case of the ASHAs we discuss in this book, the Indian state included the activists who developed the Mitanin program in Chhattisgarh that was the model for the ASHA program; the officials who, eager to reach the Sustainable Development Goals (SDGs), decided to give incentives to ASHAs for specific outcomes like women giving birth at health facilities; the committed high-level government policymakers and researchers who created the activism training modules focusing on health rights and women's rights; the state and district level supervisors who decided, in practice, not to train ASHAs as activists for those rights; the overwhelmed nurses and Auxiliary Nurse-Midwives who pushed some of their own work onto the ASHAs; the *gram panchayat* of elected officials who selected ASHAs through political processes; the politically connected union leaders who sometimes promoted ASHA interests and sometimes did not; and, of course, the ASHAs themselves. As this book has shown, each one of these groups of actors shaped the ASHA program, sometimes in unexpected ways.

Here, we join other anthropologists in calling for attention to complexity when discussing and analyzing the effects of global health programs.[11] The ways that global health programs are conceptualized, and the ways they operate in the world, are multifaceted. This means that discussions of phenomena like biopower, governmentality, and biosecurity—common frames in the anthropological literature on global health projects—need to be multifaceted too. We agree with Joao Biehl that the way forward in this space is to embrace "ethnographic ambiguities and the complexities of how projects are actually conceptualized, implemented, and worked out, or desired by people themselves."[12] Understanding how power works in global health programs requires deep and thoughtful ethnographic attention to the unexpected dynamics that proliferate when policies actually play out in practice.[13]

Anthropological work can thrive in these spaces of complexity. Our methods and our writing conventions embrace the ways that the world is surprising and complicated. And it is through this attention to nuance and detail that meaningful change can happen.

Promoting ASHA Voices

As far as how to achieve that change, we do have some ideas. One thing became extraordinarily clear to us in the process of writing this book: there is enormous, under-appreciated potential in Rajasthan's ASHAs. As a group, they are committed, funny, intelligent, and above all courageous, and as they have grown into their work in the past ten years, they have developed an appetite for re-shaping the world around them.

As they were not slow to point out to us, Rajasthan's ASHAs are intimately familiar with every child at every house in this state of more than seventy million people. Yet, although the shifts in their positions at home over the past ten years are striking, ASHAs had much more trouble finding a voice within the health system. In general terms, the health system was slow to recognize them as worthy of pay and benefits; slow to ask for their insights and not just for their data; and quick to criticize their mistakes.

In this capacity, Rajasthan's particular health system was similar to most around the world. CHWs consistently struggle to gain appreciation for the value of their work and their insights.[14] Gurha Sajjanpura's ASHAs, like many CHWs globally, occupied the lowest rung of a bureaucracy that frequently treated them as labor to be trained and disciplined, rather than as experts in the health of their communities.[15] Across CHW programs around the world, the extremely low pay and top-down nature of directives and accountability, along with the fact that female CHWs are expected to convince their neighbors to comply with the demands of the state, limit the degree to which CHWs can work to improve health in transformative ways.[16]

In this sense, the story of ASHAs in Rajasthan is not just a story about ASHAs in Rajasthan; rather, it is a story about how we think and talk about the contributions of women in rural communities—as whether they are seen as worthy of wages, respect, and advancement, and as worthy of having a seat at the policy table.

To this end, we have a few recommendations—for the ASHA program, but also for CHW programs in general.

1. Provide secure employment and a living wage for CHWs.

What the ASHAs we worked with—and their families—wanted above all else was very clear. They wanted a permanent government position, with a living wage and benefits. These were what Meena, Anita, and Seema were fighting for, and with good reason. Many women were attempting to support their families through their work. But even if they were not, for nearly all ASHAs the possibility of these benefits at some point in the future was central to taking the work at all. The ASHA program in Rajasthan was, like the ASHAs themselves, running on hope: it was successfully harnessing ASHAs' labor because the ASHAs hoped that one day this job will lead to something more.

Providing that something more is probably essential to a robust, successful, long-term program. As a recent Women in Global Health report argued, "health systems are weakened by depending on women's unpaid work."[17] Unpaid and underpaid health work is mostly carried out by women, globally and in India, and both reflects and reinforces gender inequality.[18] World Health Organization policy is that CHW work should be decent work, with fair remuneration for the extent of work a CHW is expected to contribute.[19]

A living wage for CHWs could have profound effects. If the *hope* of having secure employment was enough to give young women in rural Rajasthan mobility, family support, and even motor scooters, what would happen if they actually had such secure employment? The shifts in gender relations could be significant, especially over the long term.

2. Create career advancement pathways for CHWs.

Another piece of the something more that ASHAs hoped for was the opportunity for further training and advancement. As Anita noted, many ASHAs had extensive experience doing midwifery and nursing tasks. Many ASHAs had, in practice, been doing the paperwork associated with these positions for years. Yet there was no career progression pathway for ASHAs to move into these salaried, regularized positions.

This is not only frustrating for ASHAs; it is a lost opportunity for the Indian health system. Unlike nurses or ANMs, all of whom commuted into Gurha Sajjanpura from a larger city, ASHAs are rooted in their communities. They understand the needs of local women deeply, and they know those women personally. Years of ASHA work give these workers an unparalleled knowledge of the health challenges their neighbors face.

Giving ASHAs career advancement opportunities, including time off and funding for gaining the education needed for higher-level positions, could root the Indian health system in rural communities in a profound way, creating a primary health system more closely tied to and attuned to the needs of rural women. The ASHAs in Gurha Sajjanpura, many of whom already have master's degrees, are ready for these steps.

One key opportunity here is giving ASHAs the opportunity to train as Community Health Officers, the new cadre of village-level health providers currently being rolled out across India. For ASHAs to move into the Community Health Officer role would require several years of advanced education in most cases. But other CHW models globally, including in low-income settings, illustrate that this is very much possible. For example, Ethiopia's Health Extension Program has successfully implemented a model of a one-year basic training for CHWs, followed by a 1,600-hour advancement training, leading to a higher-level CHW. We are not suggesting this exact model be replicated in India. But it does illustrate that long-term education for rural CHWs is eminently possible in low-income contexts.

Community Health Officers and ANMs serve the same population as ASHAs, but with an expanded skillset. If ASHAs who have served an area for years are given the opportunity to advance their skills and bring that expanded knowledge back as Community Health Officers or ANMs, building on their existing deep community knowledge gained over years of service as an ASHA, it would be a powerful combination perhaps unparalleled in any health system currently in existence.

3. Create structures to protect CHWs from harassment and exploitation, and make absolutely sure those structures are robust and operational.

Some ASHAs we spoke to had troubling experiences of harassment and exploitation by supervisors. This was not so much the case in Gurha Sajjanpura, where supervisory structures were relatively benign. And there are wonderful supervisors within the Indian health system working tirelessly to serve communities. But the fact remains that many ASHAs experience harassment and exploitation, ranging from economic harassment to sexual harassment to being asked to do a wide variety of the job responsibilities of their supervisors.[20]

This issue is not unique to the ASHA program. The issue of CHW harassment and violence is a global one, tied to the global ideologies of CHW programs discussed in Chapter 1.[21] The fact that most CHW programs are made up of women, often lower-status women, supervised by men, often higher-status men, is at the root of this issue.[22] Normalization of routine, minor harassment is a key facilitator of more serious harassment, as it can naturalize power structures that can become dangerous to women.[23]

In fact, India is a leader in protections for Community Health Workers. The gang rape of an ASHA in 2016 led to new guidelines that were proactive by global standards. There are guidelines to collect information on harassment and take action, to bring village-level accountability mechanisms to bear, and to train all staff in preventing violence against women.[24] These steps are not always carried out in practice, so focus on implementation of these profoundly useful guidelines would be beneficial.

There are also deeper solutions here—solutions which integrate beautifully with giving CHWs a living wage and opportunities for advancement. As the International Labour Organization (ILO) has observed, job security is a key determinant of workplace safety.[25] Full professionalization for CHWs could include professional protections like HR staff who can confidentially receive and investigate issues of harassment and abuse. The "volunteer" label can unfortunately sometimes mean that these protections are not present for CHWs around the world. But they are critical.

4. Support unionization by and for CHWs.

ASHAs like Anita, Seema, and Meena are intelligent, committed, and savvy. They are ready to be union leaders. But without external support and higher-power champions, they are having trouble making progress. A key role for CHW allies would be to work on facilitating these structures, to support unions by and for ASHAs (and other CHWs globally) that have the structure and the connections to move policy.

Unions in other countries have secured major gains for CHWs. In Pakistan, CHW activism has led to a permanent, regularized job for Pakistan's female CHWs.[26] Other useful examples of successful CHW organizing exist, including in Brazil and the United States.[27]

There is a need for CHWs across contexts to learn from each other about what worked in terms of labor organization—and also a need for CHWs in specific contexts to learn what has worked in other sectors locally. The creative creation of such learning exchanges could potentially facilitate CHWs in taking leadership roles within labor organizations. It could also potentially be a way that lower-income rural women gain knowledge on how to gain political power.

5. Give CHWs a seat at the policy table.

What ASHAs also wanted, in addition to being paid, was to be *heard*. Quite simply, ASHAs' deep desire to share their knowledge is what made this book possible.

Far too little policy is shaped by ASHA knowledge: their knowledge of what health issues affect their neighbors, their true connection with rural mothers, their acute awareness of what is working and not working at the ground level of health systems. Of course, paid, supported ASHAs with a career progression pathway could make the deepest contributions here.[28]

Accountability in the ASHA program has generally flowed downward, with

ASHAs' data collection, in particular, being closely scrutinized. Accountability, or even feedback, flowing upward—from CHWs to their managers or the health program itself—is rare in CHW programs.[29] Yet, many programs might function better if the needs of those actually implementing interventions were considered in program design.[30]

The ASHA program is mature enough, with a sophisticated enough workforce, that it would be an excellent place to think about models of bottom-up program design. What could we learn from this workforce of one million rural women, spread across India, about the health needs of other rural women? What can they teach us about better ways to deliver care?

ASHAs are ready to engage on these questions, if we are ready to ask.

ACKNOWLEDGMENTS

Our first and deepest thanks go to the members of the community that we call Gurha Sajjanpura in this book. The warmth and generosity of our hosts made this work a joy. We gratefully appreciate the hospitality of Shankar Lal Sain, Parvati Devi, Malu Ram Sain, Punam Fevi, Jitender Sain, and Mamta Devi, and thank the young Lakxita, Vanshika, and Gouravi for the laughter and the games. Hukum Kanwar, who makes what is unquestionably the best mango curry in India, cheerfully kept us fed. Our hosts gave us welcoming and comfortable places to stay, and even sewed a gorgeous, colorful *ghagra choli* so Svea could dress like a real Rajasthani woman. The laughter, the great food, and the family events we shared will stay with us.

Most of all, we thank the ASHAs, Anganwadi Workers, and Anganwadi Helpers—and the families of these workers—who so generously opened their homes and their lives to us. This book exists thanks to you; we are sorry it has taken us so long, and hope that it achieves just a bit of what you hoped it would.

While our work started in Gurha Sajjanpura, it did not end there. Our heartfelt thanks to Shahrukh Khan, our driver, for ensuring safe and smooth travels as well as friendly companionship throughout our work.

This project was supported through a Fulbright-Nehru Fellowship. We received additional financial support from Middlebury College and the Johns Hopkins Department of International Health. We are grateful to Johns Hopkins University for providing the funding to make this book open access.

The support we received from the Fulbright-Nehru program went far beyond funding. Priyanjana Ghosh and the exceptional staff of the United States–India Educational Foundation in Delhi were a true pleasure to work with. A particular huge thanks goes to them for introducing the two of us!

This work would not have been possible without the thoughtful input of officials in the Rajasthan Ministry of Women and Child Development. We are grateful for their permission to do this work. They bear no responsibility for what we write or the conclusions we draw in this book.

We are grateful to a number of generous scholars who read and commented on this manuscript. Marium Sultan, Jen Barr, Shalini Singh, Matt Luck, Emily Mendenhall, Anat Rosenthal, and the students in Jill Owczarczak's ethnographic methods class gave insightful feedback that helped enormously in making the book clearer. Gianna Mosser, Zack Gresham, and many others at Vanderbilt University Press also gave helpful guidance. Two anonymous peer reviewers of this manuscript also gave extremely useful suggestions that shaped the book in great ways.

Soniya Kanwar, Surendra's sister, drew the beautiful illustrations in this book. We are grateful for her collaboration, her companionship during fieldwork, and her contributions.

I am extraordinarily fortunate to have two mentors in my life who continue to provide support, encouragement, and guidance decades after they should no longer have to feel responsible for me. Judith Justice and Peter Brown have been sounding boards, sages, and friends throughout my academic life, and throughout the process of writing this book. I constantly try to be half as good to a few of my students as both of them are on a continuous basis to me.

I am enormously grateful, always, to Surendra and his family. Narayan Singh, Geeta Kanwar, and their entire family, as well as Surendra's wife Parkash, were warm and welcoming in the very best way. I'm pretty sure my experience in Rajasthan would have been very incomplete without my being pushed on a colorful swing while being devilishly encouraged to yell the name of my husband. Thank you so much for the deep gut belly laughs, and for the dance lessons.

The initial spark for this project came from a "think-in" on Community Health Workers at American University. The conversations at that meeting about the need to better understand how unionization could be a vehicle for Community Health Worker voice were the impetus for this project. My sincere thanks to Jonathan Fox, Marta Schaaf, and others at the Accountability Research Center for convening that conference and making those conversations possible, and to the conference participants, including Kerry Scott, Steph Topp, Thokozile Mercy Maboe, and Abhay Shukla, for shaping my thinking.

As the project developed, I benefited from incredibly generous guidance and insight. Kavita Bhatia has continually been a warm, smart, and informed sounding board. The entire staff of SATHI in Pune, India—and the ASHAs and union organizers they introduced me to in the state of Maharashtra—were instrumental in helping me understand the shape of ASHA training and unionization in India before this project began.

My colleagues at the Indian Institute of Health Management Research in Jaipur are an ongoing source of inspiration and knowledge. Piyusha Majumdar, S. D. Gupta, and Rahul Ghai have made IIHMR a real home, and I'm so grateful for their wisdom and their support. They have mentored me in many ways, and they are not responsible for our conclusions here.

While Surendra was untiring in moving this manuscript forward, my part of the work would likely never have been completed were it not for the support and encouragement of my Writing Accountability Group. Adam Koon, Ligia Paina, Daniela Rodriguez, Rosemary Morgan, Yusra Shawar, Connie Ho, and Andres Vecino helped me forward when I was stuck, cheered me on when I wasn't, and sent a constant stream of hilarious (and maybe even sometimes helpful) writing memes over WhatsApp. Their insistence that I reserve time for writing was essential to the completion of this book. Every writer should have a WAG as wonderful as this one, and few of us get one. I do truly hope to have them around for life.

My family's support for my work has always been enthusiastic and unwavering. My parents, Bruce and Sally Closser, have always provided me with a strong foundation of love and support. My mom would have been so proud to see this book. My son Kaif Rehman accommodated my extended absences with true generosity; I'm continuously grateful to be the parent of such a wonderful human. And it is a real gift to have a partner like Matt Luck, who came all the way to Rajasthan to meet the people I care about.

Svea

I offer a heart full of thanks to the entire Shekhawat family for their motivation and belief in me. First of all, I want to thank my Bede Mummy and Papa, the late Chagan Kanwar and late Maden Singh ji. I learned so much from them, and that will support me for a lifetime.

I thank my parents Geeta Kanwar and Narayan Singh for their unwavering support and encouragement. My mother's smile and my father's pride have been driving forces in my life.

A special thank you to my wife, Parkash, and son, Ahtharva, for being my constant sources of inspiration.

I extend my thanks to my guides and mentors, Dr. Svea Closser and Dr. Bela Kothari. Their guidance has nurtured my growth.

I am also thankful to my colleagues from the University of Rajasthan, Naveen, Ravi, and Mahesh, for their encouragement and support.

To my dear friends Alisa, Sara, Anjali, Shyam Singh, Maluram, and Chothmal, thank you for being in my life. Without all of you it is quite impossible.

Surendra

NOTES

Preface

1. Ann Grodzins Gold and Bhoju Ram Gujar, *In the Time of Trees and Sorrows: Nature, Power, and Memory in Rajasthan* (Duke University Press, 2002).

Chapter 1

1. Michelle Murphy, "The Girl: Mergers of Feminism and Finance in Neoliberal Times," *Scholar & Feminist Online*, 11, no. 1–2 (July 8, 2013), https://sfonline.barnard.edu/the-girl-mergers-of-feminism-and-finance-in-neoliberal-times.
2. Sarah Gimbel et al., "Donor Data Vacuuming," *Medicine Anthropology Theory* 5, no. 2 (May 15, 2018); Jeremy Shiffman and Yusra Ribhi Shawar, "Strengthening Accountability of the Global Health Metrics Enterprise," *Lancet* 395, no. 10234 (May 2, 2020): 1452–56.
3. Mabelle Arole and Rajanikant Arole, "A Comprehensive Rural Health Project in Jamkhed (India)," in *Health for the People*, by Kenneth W. Newell (World Health Organization, 1975), 70.
4. Henry B. Perry and Jon Rohde, "The Jamkhed Comprehensive Rural Health Project and the Alma-Ata Vision of Primary Health Care," *American Journal of Public Health* 109, no. 5 (March 21, 2019): 699–704; Mabelle Arole and Rajanikant Arole, *Jamkhed: A Comprehensive Rural Health Project* (Macmillan, 1994).
5. Arole and Arole, *Jamkhed*; Perry and Rohde, "Jamkhed Comprehensive."
6. Kenneth W. Newell, *Health by the People* (World Health Organization, 1975), x, https://apps.who.int/iris/handle/10665/40514.
7. M. Cueto, "The Origins of Primary Health Care and Selective Primary Health Care," *American Journal of Public Health* 94, no. 11 (November 1, 2004): 1864–74; S. M. Tollman, "The Pholela Health Centre—the Origins of Community-Oriented Primary Health Care (COPC)," *South African Medical Journal* 84, no. 10 (1994): 653–58.
8. M. Cueto, "Origins of Primary Health Care"; Judith Justice, *Policies, Plans, and People* (University of California Press, 1986).
9. World Health Organization, "Declaration of Alma-Ata," in *International Conference on Primary Health Care* (Alma-Ata, USSR, 1978).
10. World Health Organization, "Declaration of Alma-Ata."
11. David Werner, "The Village Health Worker: Lackey or Liberator?," *World Health Forum* 2, no. 1 (1981): 47.
12. Werner, "The Village Health Worker," 49.

13. C. Campbell and K. Scott, "Retreat from Alma Ata? The WHO's Report on Task Shifting to Community Health Workers for AIDS Care in Poor Countries," *Global Public Health* 6, no. 2 (March 1, 2011): 125–38; Christopher J. Colvin and Alison Swartz, "Extension Agents or Agents of Change?," *Annals of Anthropological Practice* 39, no. 1 (May 1, 2015): 29–41; Kenneth Maes, "Community Health Workers and Social Change," *Annals of Anthropological Practice* 39, no. 1 (May 1, 2015): 1–15; Gill Walt and Lucy Gilson, *Community Health Workers in National Programmes: Just Another Pair of Hands?* (Open University Press, 1990).

14. Debabar Banerji, "Politics of Rural Health in India," *International Journal of Health Services* 35, no. 4 (October 1, 2005): 783–96.

15. Banerji, "Politics of Rural Health."

16. Charles Leslie, "What Caused India's Massive Community Health Workers Scheme: A Sociology of Knowledge," *Social Science & Medicine* 21, no. 8 (January 1, 1985): 923–30.

17. Mark A. Nichter, "The Primary Health Center as a Social System: PHC, Social Status, and the Issue of Team-Work in South Asia," *Social Science & Medicine* 23, no. 4 (January 1, 1986): 349.

18. Rushikesh Maru, "Community Health Worker: Some Aspects of the Experience at the National Level," *Medico Friend Circle Bulletin*, March 1980, 3.

19. Leslie, "What Caused India's."

20. Nichter, "Primary Health Center"; Ashish Bose, *Studies in Social Dynamics of Primary Health Care* (Hindustan Publishing Corporation, 1983).

21. Kavita Bhatia, "Community Health Worker Programs in India: A Rights-Based Review," *Perspectives in Public Health* 134, no. 5 (2014): 276–82.

22. James Pfeiffer, "International NGOs in the Mozambique Health Sector: The 'Velvet Glove' of Privatization," in *Unhealthy Health Policy* (AltaMira Press, 2004); J. Y. Kim et al., eds., *Dying for Growth: Global Inequality and the Health of the Poor* (Common Courage Press, 2002).

23. Susan B. Rifkin, "Alma Ata after 40 Years: Primary Health Care and Health for All—from Consensus to Complexity," *BMJ Global Health* 3, no. 3 (December 1, 2018): e001188; Beth A. Uzwiak and Siobhan Curran, "Gendering the Burden of Care: Health Reform and the Paradox of Community Participation in Western Belize," *Medical Anthropology Quarterly* 30, no. 1 (2016): 100–121.

24. Banerji, "Politics of Rural Health."

25. Diana Bowser et al., "A Cost-Effectiveness Analysis of Community Health Workers in Mozambique," *Journal of Primary Care & Community Health* 6, no. 4 (October 1, 2015): 227–32; Andy Haines et al., "Achieving Child Survival Goals: Potential Contribution of Community Health Workers," *The Lancet* 369, no. 9579 (2007): 2121–31; Kelsey Vaughan et al., "Costs and Cost-Effectiveness of Community Health Workers: Evidence from a Literature Review," *Human Resources for Health* 13, no. 1 (September 1, 2015): 71.

26. Justice, *Policies, Plans, and People*.

27. James Pfeiffer and Mark Nichter, "What Can Critical Medical Anthropology Contribute to Global Health?," *Medical Anthropology Quarterly* 22, no. 4 (December 2008): 410–15.

28. Katerini Storeng, "Politics and Practices of Global Health: Critical Ethnographies of Health Systems," *Global Public Health* 9, no. 8 (September 14, 2014): 858–64.

29. "The Ethnographic Lens," in *Health Policy and Systems Research: A Methodology Reader*, by Lucy Gilson (World Health Organization, 2012), 235–52.

30. Claire Wendland, *A Heart for the Work: Journeys Through an African Medical School* (University of Chicago Press, 2010); Julie Livingston, *Improvising Medicine: An African Oncology Ward in an Emerging Cancer Epidemic* (Duke University Press, 2012).

31. Ruth Prince and Hannah Brown, eds., *Volunteer Economies: The Politics and Ethics of Voluntary Labour in Africa* (James Currey, 2016); Svea Closser et al., "Per Diems in Polio Eradication: Perspectives From Community Health Workers and Officials," *American Journal of Public Health* 107, no. 9 (September 2017): 1470–76; Hannah Brown and Ruth J. Prince, "Introduction: Volunteer Labor—Pasts and Futures of Work, Development, and Citizenship in East Africa," *African Studies Review* 58, no. 02 (September 2015): 29–42; Kerry Scott and Shobhit Shanker, "Tying Their Hands?: Institutional Obstacles to the Success of the ASHA Community Health Worker Programme in Rural North India," *AIDS Care* 22, no. suppl. 2 (2010): 1606–12.

32. Closser et al., "Per Diems in Polio Eradication"; Svea Closser and Rashid Jooma, "Why We Must Provide Better Support for Pakistan's Female Frontline Health Workers," *PLoS Med* 10, no. 10 (October 8, 2013): e1001528; Ippolytos Kalofonos, "'All They Do Is Pray': Community Labour and the Narrowing of 'Care' during Mozambique's HIV Scale-Up," *Global Public Health* 9, no. 1–2 (February 12, 2014): 7–24; Kenneth Maes, "Volunteerism or Labor Exploitation? Harnessing the Volunteer Spirit to Sustain AIDS Treatment Programs in Urban Ethiopia," *Human Organization* 71, no. 1 (January 1, 2012): 54–64; Zara Trafford, Alison Swartz, and Christopher J. Colvin, "'Contract to Volunteer': South African Community Health Worker Mobilization for Better Labor Protection," *NEW SOLUTIONS: A Journal of Environmental and Occupational Health Policy* 27, no. 4 (February 1, 2018): 648–66.

33. Rifkin, "Alma Ata after 40 Years"; Uzwiak and Curran, "Gendering the Burden"; Closser et al., "Per Diems in Polio Eradication"; James Wintrup, "Health by the People, Again? The Lost Lessons of Alma-Ata in a Community Health Worker Programme in Zambia," in "Health for all? Pasts, Presents and Futures of Universal Health Care and Universal Health Coverage," special issue of *Social Science & Medicine*, 319 (February 1, 2023): 115257.

34. Closser and Jooma, "Why We Must"; Kenneth Maes et al., "Psychosocial Distress among Unpaid Community Health Workers in Rural Ethiopia: Comparing Leaders in Ethiopia's Women's Development Army to Their Peers," *Social Science & Medicine* 230 (June 1, 2019): 138–46; Kenneth Maes and Ippolytos Kalofonos, "Becoming and Remaining Community Health Workers: Perspectives from Ethiopia and Mozambique," *Social Science & Medicine* 87 (June 1, 2013): 52–59; Prince and Brown, *Volunteer Economies*.

35. Svea Closser et al., "Political Connections and Psychosocial Wellbeing among Women's Development Army Leaders in Rural Amhara, Ethiopia: Towards a Holistic Understanding of Community Health Workers' Socioeconomic Status," *Social Science & Medicine* 266 (December 1, 2020): 113373; Kenneth Maes, *The Lives of Community Health Workers: Local Labor and Global Health in Urban Ethiopia* (Routledge, 2016); Prince and Brown, *Volunteer Economies*; Svea Closser, "'I Need Money, That's the Only Reason I Do It': Youth 'Volunteers,' Unemployment, and International Action in Pakistan's Health Sector," in *The Crisis in Global Youth Unemployment*, ed. T. Mayer, Sujata Moorti, and Jamie McCallum (Routledge, 2018), 57–75; Catherine van de Ruit, "Unintended Consequences of Community Health Worker Programs in South Africa," *Qualitative Health Research* 29, no. 11 (September 1, 2019): 1535–48.

36. Closser, "'I Need Money"; Closser et al., "Political Connections."

37. Claire Glenton et al., "The Female Community Health Volunteer Programme in Nepal: Decision Makers' Perceptions of Volunteerism, Payment and Other Incentives," *Social Science & Medicine* 70, no. 12 (June 2010): 1920–27.

38. Kenneth C. Maes, Brandon A. Kohrt, and Svea Closser, "Culture, Status and Context in Community Health Worker Pay: Pitfalls and Opportunities for Policy Research. A Commentary on Glenton et al. (2010)," *Social Science & Medicine* 71, no. 8 (October 2010): 1375–78; Kenneth Maes, "'Volunteers Are Not Paid Because They Are Priceless': Community Health Worker Capacities and Values in an AIDS Treatment Intervention in Urban Ethiopia," *Medical Anthropology Quarterly* 29, no. 1 (2015): 97–115.

39. Alex M. Nading, "Dengue Mosquitoes Are Single Mothers: Biopolitics Meets Ecological Aesthetics in Nicaraguan Community Health Work," *Cultural Anthropology* 27, no. 4 (2012): 572–96.

40. Maes, *Lives of Community Health Workers*, 2016; Maes, "Volunteerism or Labor Exploitation?"; Kenneth Maes, Svea Closser, and Ippolytos Kalofonos, "Listening to Community Health Workers: How Ethnographic Research Can Inform Positive Relationships Among Community Health Workers, Health Institutions, and Communities," *American Journal of Public Health* 104, no. 5 (May 2014): e5–9; Maes and Kalofonos, "Becoming and Remaining"; Alison Swartz and Christopher J. Colvin, "'It's in Our Veins': Caring Natures and Material Motivations of Community Health Workers in Contexts of Economic Marginalisation," *Critical Public Health* 25, no. 2 (July 30, 2014): 1–14; Uzwiak and Curran, "Gendering the Burden."

41. H. B. Perry, R. Zulliger, and M. M. Rogers, "Community Health Workers in Low-, Middle-, and High-Income Countries: An Overview of Their History, Recent Evolution, and Current Effectiveness," *Annual Review of Public Health* 35 (2014): 399–421; One Million Community Health Workers Campaign, "One Million Community Health Workers Map," 2018, http://1millionhealthworkers.org/operations-room-map.

42. World Health Organization, "Delivered by Women, Led by Men: A Gender and Equity Analysis of the Global Health and Social Workforce" (World Health Organization, 2019), http://www.who.int/hrh/resources/health-observer24/en/.

43. "One Million Community Health Workers: Technical Task Force Report" (Earth Institute at Columbia University, 2013), http://1millionhealthworkers.org/files/2013/01/1mCHW_TechnicalTaskForceReport.pdf.

44. Olagoke Akintola, "Unpaid HIV/AIDS–Care in Southern Africa: Forms, Context, and Implications," *Feminist Economics* 14, no. 4 (2008): 117; Sylvia Chant, "The 'Feminisation of Poverty' and the 'Feminisation' of Anti-Poverty Programmes: Room for Revision?," *Journal of Development Studies* 44, no. 2 (February 2008): 165–97; Sylvia Chant, "Women, Girls and World Poverty: Empowerment, Equality or Essentialism?," *International Development Planning Review* 38, no. 1 (2016): 1–24; Greta Friedemann-Sánchez and Joan M. Griffin, "Defining the Boundaries between Unpaid Labor and Unpaid Caregiving: Review of the Social and Health Sciences Literature," *Journal of Human Development and Capabilities* 12, no. 4 (November 1, 2011): 511–34; Maxine Molyneux, "Mothers at the Service of the New Poverty Agenda: Progresa/Oportunidades, Mexico's Conditional Transfer Programme," *Social Policy & Administration* 40, no. 4 (2006): 425–49; Jesus Ramirez-Valles, "Promoting Health, Promoting Women: The Construction of Female

and Professional Identities in the Discourse of Community Health Workers," *Social Science & Medicine* 47, no. 11 (December 1998): 1749–62; Aradhana Sharma, "Crossbreeding Institutions, Breeding Struggle: Women's Empowerment, Neoliberal Governmentality, and State (Re)Formation in India," *Cultural Anthropology* 21, no. 1 (2006): 60–95.

45. María Puig de la Bellacasa, "'Nothing Comes Without Its World': Thinking with Care," *Sociological Review* 60, no. 2 (2012): 197–216; Ramirez-Valles, "Promoting Health."

46. de la Bellacasa, "'Nothing Comes Without Its World.'"

47. Joan C. Tronto, *Caring Democracy: Markets, Equality, and Justice* (New York University Press, 2013), 31.

48. Tronto, *Caring Democracy*.

49. Patricia Kingori, Francis Kombe, and Alexandra Fehr, "Making Global Health 'Work': Frontline Workers' Labour in Research and Interventions," *Global Public Health* 17, no. 12 (December 2, 2022): 4077–86.

50. Anna Kalbarczyk et al., "A Light Touch Intervention with a Heavy Lift—Gender, Space and Risk in a Global Vaccination Programme," *Global Public Health* 17, no. 12 (July 18, 2022): 1–14; Asha S. George et al., "Violence against Female Health Workers Is Tip of Iceberg of Gender Power Imbalances," *BMJ* 371 (October 27, 2020): m3546.

51. Svea Closser et al., "Breaking the Silence on Gendered Harassment and Assault of Community Health Workers: An Analysis of Ethnographic Studies," *BMJ Global Health* 8, no. 5 (May 1, 2023): e011749; Lavanya Rao et al., "Investigating Violence against Accredited Social Health Activists (ASHAs): A Mixed Methods Study from Rural North Karnataka, India," *Journal of Global Health Reports* 5 (June 18, 2021): e2021054.

52. Svea Closser, "Pakistan's Lady Health Worker Labor Movement and the Moral Economy of Heroism," *Annals of Anthropological Practice* 39, no. 1 (May 1, 2015): 16–28.

53. Closser et al., "Per Diems in Polio Eradication."

54. "One Million Community Health Workers: Technical Task Force Report."

55. Roosa Sofia Tikkanen et al., "An Anthropological History of Nepal's Female Community Health Volunteer Program: Gender, Policy, and Social Change," *International Journal for Equity in Health* 23, no. 1 (April 13, 2024): 70; Bhatia, "Community Health Worker."

56. T. Sundararaman, "Universalisation of ICDS and Community Health Worker Programmes: Lessons from Chhattisgarh," *Economic and Political Weekly* 41, no. 34 (2006): 3674–79.

57. Suchi Pande, "Community Health Workers as Rights Defenders: The Mitanin Experience in India," *Development in Practice* 33, no 8 (2023): 939–44.

58. Schaaf et al., "Report on the 'Think-in.'"

59. Binayak Sen, "Myth of the Mitanin: Political Constraints on Structural Reforms in Healthcare in Chhattisgarh," *Medico Friend Circle Bulletin* 311 (2005): 12–17.

60. Samir Garg and Suchi Pande, "Learning to Sustain Change: Mitanin Community Health Workers Promote Public Accountability in India" (Accountability Research Center, August 2018).

61. Closser et al., "Per Diems"; Rifkin, "Alma Ata after 40 Years."

62. J Hanefeld and M Musheke, "What Impact Do Global Health Initiatives Have on Human Resources for Antiretroviral Treatment Roll-out? A Qualitative Policy Analysis of Implementation Processes in Zambia.," *Human Resources for Health* 7, no. 8 (2009).

63. Sujay R Joshi and Matthew George, "Healthcare through Community Participation:

Role of ASHAs," *Economic and Political Weekly* 47, no. 10 (2012): 70–76; Scott and Shanker, "Tying Their Hands?"; Vincanne Adams, *Metrics: What Counts in Global Health* (Duke University Press, 2016); Elsa Fan and Elanah Uretsky, "In Search of Results: Anthropological Interrogations of Evidence-Based Global Health," *Critical Public Health* 27, no. 2 (2017): 157–62.

64. Arima Mishra, "'Trust and Teamwork Matter': Community Health Workers' Experiences in Integrated Service Delivery in India," *Global Public Health* 9, no. 8 (September 14, 2014): 960–74.

65. Amy Cooper, "What Does Health Activism Mean in Venezuela's Barrio Adentro Program? Understanding Community Health Work in Political and Cultural Context," *Annals of Anthropological Practice* 39, no. 1 (2015): 58–72.

66. Kenneth Maes et al., "Using Community Health Workers," *Annals of Anthropological Practice* 39, no. 1 (May 1, 2015): 42–57.

67. Sidsel Roalkvam, "Health Governance in India: Citizenship as Situated Practice," *Global Public Health* 9, no. 8 (2014): 910–26.

68. Committee on Empowerment of Women (2010–2011), Fifteenth Lok Sabha, "Eleventh Report: Working Conditions of ASHAs" (New Delhi: Lok Sabha Secretariat, September 2011).

69. Alex M. Nading, "'Love Isn't There in Your Stomach,'" *Medical Anthropology Quarterly* 27, no. 1 (2013): 84–102; Ryan I. Logan, "'A Poverty in Understanding': Assessing the Structural Challenges Experienced by Community Health Workers and Their Clients," *Global Public Health* 15, no. 1 (January 2, 2020): 137–50.

70. Jonathan N. Maupin, "Shifting Identities," *Annals of Anthropological Practice* 39, no. 1 (2015): 73–88; Alison Swartz, "Legacy, Legitimacy, and Possibility," *Medical Anthropology Quarterly* 27, no. 2 (2013): 139–54.

71. Colvin and Swartz, "Extension Agents."

72. Maes, *Lives of Community Health Workers*, 2016; Maes, "Volunteerism or Labor Exploitation?"

73. Kerry Scott, Asha S. George, and Rajani R. Ved, "Taking Stock of 10 Years of Published Research on the ASHA Programme: Examining India's National Community Health Worker Programme from a Health Systems Perspective," *Health Research Policy and Systems* 17, no. 1 (March 25, 2019): 29.

74. Cecilie Nordfeldt and Sidsel Roalkvam, "Choosing Vaccination: Negotiating Child Protection and Good Citizenship in Modern India," *Forum for Development Studies* 37, no. 3 (November 1, 2010): 327–47; Reetu Sharma, Premila Webster, and Sanghita Bhattacharyya, "Factors Affecting the Performance of Community Health Workers in India: A Multi-Stakeholder Perspective," *Global Health Action* 7 (October 13, 2014).

75. Nordfeldt and Roalkvam, "Choosing Vaccination," 344.

76. Sharma, Webster, and Bhattacharyya, "Factors Affecting the Performance."

77. Kavita Bhatia, "Performance-Based Incentives of the ASHA Scheme: Stakeholders' Perspectives," *Economic and Political Weekly* 49, no. 22 (2014): 145–51, http://www.jstor.org/stable/24479649.

78. Trafford, Swartz, and Colvin, "'Contract to Volunteer'"; Closser, "Pakistan's Lady Health Worker."

79. Tikkanen et al., "An Anthropological History"; Catherine van de Ruit and Alexandra

Breckenridge, "South African Community Health Workers' Pursuit of Occupational Security," *Gender, Work & Organization* 31, no. 4 (2022), 1560–81.

80. van de Ruit and Breckenridge, "South African Community."

81. Ramah McKay, "Global Health's Durable Dreams: Ethnography, 'Community Health Workers' and Health without Health Infrastructure," *Africa* 90, no. 1 (January 2020): 95–111.

82. Paul Farmer et al., *Reimagining Global Health: An Introduction* (University of California Press, 2013); M. D. Salmaan Keshavjee, *Blind Spot: How Neoliberalism Infiltrated Global Health* (University of California Press, 2014); João Biehl, "Theorizing Global Health," *Medicine Anthropology Theory* 3, no. 2 (September 13, 2016).

83. Svea Closser et al., "The Anthropology of Health Systems: A History and Review," in "Health Systems Performance or Performing Health Systems?," special issue of *Social Science & Medicine* 300 (May 1, 2022): 114314.

Chapter 2

1. Ann Gold, "Purdah Is as Purdah's Kept," in *Listen to the Heron's Words*, ed. Gloria Raheja and Ann Gold (University of California Press, 1994), 164–81.

2. Patricia Kingori and René Gerrets, "The Masking and Making of Fieldworkers and Data in Postcolonial Global Health Research Contexts," *Critical Public Health* 29, no. 4 (August 8, 2019): 494–507.

3. Cal (Crystal) Biruk, "Capture-Recapture," *American Ethnologist* 49, no. 4 (2022): 549–62.

4. Eleanor Hutchinson et al., "Data Value and Care Value in the Practice of Health Systems: A Case Study in Uganda," *Social Science & Medicine* 211 (August 1, 2018): 123–30.

5. Svea Closser, *Chasing Polio in Pakistan: Why the World's Largest Public Health Initiative May Fail* (Vanderbilt University Press, 2010); James C. Scott, *Weapons of the Weak* (Yale University Press, 1985).

6. Kingori and Gerrets, "The Masking and Making."

7. Patricia Kingori and René Gerrets, "Morals, Morale and Motivations in Data Fabrication: Medical Research Fieldworkers Views and Practices in Two Sub-Saharan African Contexts," *Social Science & Medicine* 166 (October 1, 2016): 150–59.

8. N. Hélène Sawadogo et al., "Promises and Perils of Mobile Health in Burkina Faso," *The Lancet* 398, no. 10302 (August 28, 2021): 738–39; Willem A. Odendaal et al., "Health Workers' Perceptions and Experiences of Using mHealth Technologies to Deliver Primary Healthcare Services: A Qualitative Evidence Synthesis," *Cochrane Database of Systematic Reviews*, no. 3 (2020).

9. S Erikson, "Global Health Business: The Production and Performativity of Statistics in Sierra Leone and Germany," *Medical Anthropology* 31, no. 4 (2012): 367–84; Robert Lorway, "Making Global Health Knowledge: Documents, Standards, and Evidentiary Sovereignty in HIV Interventions in South India," *Critical Public Health* 27, no. 2 (March 15, 2017): 177–92; Elanah Uretsky, "'We Can't Do That Here': Negotiating Evidence in HIV Prevention Campaigns in Southwest China," *Critical Public Health* 27, no. 2 (March 15, 2017): 205–16.

10. Elsa L. Fan, "Counting Results: Performance-Based Financing and HIV Testing among MSM in China," *Critical Public Health* 27, no. 2 (March 15, 2017): 217–27; Hutchinson et al., "Data Value and Care Value."

Chapter 3

1. Arole and Arole, *Jamkhed*; Sulakshana Nandi and Helen Schneider, "Addressing the Social Determinants of Health: A Case Study from the Mitanin (Community Health Worker) Programme in India," *Health Policy and Planning* 29, no. suppl 2 (September 1, 2014): ii71–81.

2. Kalofonos, "'All They Do Is Pray'"; Maes, "'Volunteers Are Not Paid'"; Nading, "'Love Isn't There.'"

3. Henrike Donner, "'The Girls Are Alright': Beauty Work and Neoliberal Regimes of Responsibility among Young Women in Urban India," *Critique of Anthropology* 43, no. 4 (December 1, 2023): 399–421; Maria Mies, "Dynamics of Sexual Division of Labour and Capital Accumulation: Women Lace Workers of Narsapur," *Economic and Political Weekly* 16, no. 10/12 (March 1981): 487–500.

4. Ann Gold, "New Light in the House: Schooling Girls in Rural North India," in *Everyday Life in South Asia*, ed. Diane Mines and Sarah Lamb (Indiana University Press, 2002), 86–99.

5. Gloria Goodwin Raheja and Ann Grodzins Gold, *Listen to the Heron's Words: Reimagining Gender and Kinship in North India* (University of California Press, 1994); Patricia Jeffery and Roger Jeffery, "Killing My Heart's Desire: Education and Female Autonomy in Rural North India," in *Women as Subjects: South Asian Histories*, ed. Nita Kumar (University Press of Virginia, 1994), 125–71.

6. Geert De Neve, "'Keeping It in the Family': Work, Education and Gender Hierarchies among Tiruppur's Industrial Capitalists," in *Being Middle-Class in India* (Routledge, 2011); Filippo Osella and Caroline Osella, "From Transience to Immanence: Consumption, Life-Cycle and Social Mobility in Kerala, South India," *Modern Asian Studies* 33, no. 4 (October 1999): 989–1020.

7. Rajni Palriwala and N. Neetha, "Care Arrangements and Bargains: Anganwadi and Paid Domestic Workers in India," *International Labour Review* 149, no. 4 (2010): 513.

8. Mies, "Dynamics of Sexual Division," 491.

9. See also R. Ved et al., "How Are Gender Inequalities Facing India's One Million ASHAs Being Addressed? Policy Origins and Adaptations for the World's Largest All-Female Community Health Worker Programme," *Human Resources for Health* 17, no. 1 (January 8, 2019): 3.

10. Padmini Swaminathan, "The Formal Creation of Informality, and Therefore, Gender Injustice: Illustrations from India's Social Sector.," *Indian Journal of Labour Economics* 58 (2015): 23–42.

Chapter 5

1. Sarah Besky, "Can a Plantation Be Fair? Paradoxes and Possibilities in Fair Trade Darjeeling Tea Certification," *Anthropology of Work Review* 29, no. 1 (2008): 1–9; Rina Agarwala, "Reshaping the Social Contract: Emerging Relations between the State and Informal Labor in India," *Theory and Society* 37, no. 4 (August 1, 2008): 375–408.

2. Kiran Saxena, "The Hindu Trade Union Movement in India: The Bharatiya Mazdoor Sangh," *Asian Survey* 33, no. 7 (1993): 685–96; Agarwala, "Reshaping the Social Contract."

3. Sarath Davala, "Independent Trade Unionism in West Bengal," *Economic and Political Weekly* 31, no. 52 (1996): L44–49.

4. Manuela Ciotti, "At the Margins of Feminist Politics? A Comparative Analysis of Women

in Dalit Politics and Hindu Right Organisations in Northern India," *Contemporary South Asia* 15, no. 4 (December 1, 2006): 437–52; Kenneth Nielsen, "Women's Activism in the Singur Movement, West Bengal," in *Women, Gender and Everyday Social Transformation in India*, ed. Anne Waldrop and Kenneth Nielsen (Anthem Press, 2014), 203–18.

5. Leela Fernandes, "Culture, Structure and Working Class Politics," *Economic and Political Weekly* 33, no. 52 (1998): L53–60; Panchali Ray, "Women in/and Trade Unions: Consciousness, Agency, and (Im)Possibilities of Alliances amongst Nurses and Attendants in Kolkata," *Contemporary South Asia* 27, no. 4 (October 2, 2019): 502–15.

6. Ray, "Women in/and Trade Unions."

7. Jonathan Parry, "Company and Contract Labour in a Central Indian Steel Plant," *Economy and Society* 42, no. 3 (August 1, 2013): 348–74; Supriya RoyChowdhury, "Old Classes and New Spaces: Urban Poverty, Unorganised Labour and New Unions," *Economic and Political Weekly* 38, no. 50 (2003): 5277–84; Andrew Sanchez and Christian Strümpell, "Sons of Soil, Sons of Steel: Autochthony, Descent and the Class Concept in Industrial India," *Modern Asian Studies* 48, no. 5 (September 2014): 1276–1301; Mark Holmström, *Industry and Inequality: The Social Anthropology of Indian Labour* (Cambridge University Press, 1984).

8. Holmström, *Industry and Inequality*, 167.

9. Andrew Sanchez, "Questioning Success: Dispossession and the Criminal Entrepreneur in Urban India," *Critique of Anthropology* 32, no. 4 (December 1, 2012): 435–57; Andrew Sanchez, *Criminal Capital: Violence, Corruption and Class in Industrial India* (Routledge, 2016).

10. Besky, "Can a Plantation"; Holmström, *Industry and Inequality*.

Chapter 6

1. Sumegha Asthana and Kaveri Mayra, "India's One Million Accredited Social Health Activists (ASHA) Win the Global Health Leaders Award at the 75th World Health Assembly: Time to Move beyond Rhetoric to Action?," *The Lancet Regional Health—Southeast Asia* 3 (August 1, 2022).

2. Priyali Prakash, "Explained | All about India's ASHA Workers, Recipients of WHO's Global Leaders Award," *The Hindu*, May 28, 2022, sec. India, https://www.thehindu.com/news/national/explained-all-about-indias-asha-workers-recipients-of-whos-global-leaders-award/article65457663.ece.

Conclusion

1. World Health Organization, "Delivered by Women."

2. Sharma, "Crossbreeding Institutions."

3. Donner, "'The Girls Are Alright.'"

4. Lamia Karim, "NGOs, State and Neoliberal Development in South Asia: The Paradigmatic Case of Bangladesh in a Global Perspective," in *Routledge Handbook of Gender in South Asia* (Routledge, 2021), 289–302.

5. Fan, "Counting Results"; Raphael Frankfurter, "Conjuring Biosecurity in the Post-Ebola Kissi Triangle: The Magic of Paperwork in a Frontier Clinic," *Medical Anthropology Quarterly* 33, no. 4 (2019): 517–38; Hutchinson et al., "Data Value."

6. Marlee Tichenor, "Data Performativity, Performing Health Work: Malaria and Labor in Senegal," *Medical Anthropology* 36, no. 5 (2017): 436–48; Diane Duclos et al., "Envisioning, Evaluating and Co-Enacting Performance in Global Health Interventions: Ethnographic Insights from Senegal," *Anthropology in Action* 26, no. 1 (2019): 21–30; Fan, "Counting Results"; Lorway, "Making Global Health Knowledge"; Uretsky, "'We Can't Do That Here.'"

7. Mishra, "'Trust and Teamwork Matter.'"

8. Adeola Oni-Orisan, "The Obligation to Count," in *Metrics*, by Vincanne Adams (Duke University Press, 2016), 82–101; Mishra, "'Trust and Teamwork Matter'"; Erikson, "Global Health Business"; Svea Closser, "The Corruption Game: Health Systems, International Agencies, and the State in South Asia," *Medical Anthropology Quarterly* 34, no. 2 (2020): 268–85.

9. Akhil Gupta, *Red Tape: Bureaucracy, Structural Violence, and Poverty in India* (Duke University Press, 2012).

10. Hutchinson et al., "Data Value"; Adams, *Metrics*.

11. Katherine Mason, *Infectious Change* (Stanford University Press, 2016); Closser et al., "Anthropology of Health Systems."

12. Biehl, "Theorizing Global Health."

13. Margaret Lock and Vinh-Kim Nguyen, *An Anthropology of Biomedicine* (John Wiley & Sons, 2011), 19; Arthur Kleinman, "Four Social Theories for Global Health," *Lancet* 375, no. 9725 (2010): 1518–19.

14. Svea Closser et al., "Does Volunteer Community Health Work Empower Women? Evidence from Ethiopia's Women's Development Army," *Health Policy and Planning* 34, no. 4 (May 1, 2019): 298–306; Colvin and Swartz, "Extension Agents"; Kenneth Maes, *The Lives of Community Health Workers: Local Labor and Global Health in Urban Ethiopia* (Routledge, 2016); Kalofonos, "'All They Do Is Pray.'"

15. Judith Justice, "Can Socio-Cultural Information Improve Health Planning? A Case Study of Nepal's Assistant Nurse-Midwife," *Social Science & Medicine* 19, no. 3 (1984): 193–98; Lynn M. Morgan, *Community Participation in Health: The Politics of Primary Care in Costa Rica* (Cambridge University Press, 1993); Nichter, "Primary Health Center"; Closser et al., "Does Volunteer Community."

16. Closser et al., "Does Volunteer Community"; Roalkvam, "Health Governance in India."

17. Women in Global Health, "Subsidizing Global Health: Women's Unpaid Work in Health Systems" (Women in Global Health, 2022), 26, https://womeningh.org/wp-content/uploads/2022/07/Pay-Women-Report-July-7-Release.pdf.

18. Jashodhara Dasgupta and Kanika Jha Kingra, "Women Workers at the Forefront of COVID-19: A Roadmap for Recovery and Resilience in India," in *The Political Economy of Post-COVID Life and Work in the Global South: Pandemic and Precarity*, ed. Sandya Hewamanne and Smytta Yadav, International Political Economy Series (Cham: Springer International Publishing, 2022), 105–31, https://doi.org/10.1007/978-3-030-93228-2_6.

19. World Health Organization, "WHO Guideline on Health Policy and System Support to Optimize Community Health Worker Programmes" (World Health Organization, 2018).

20. Rao et al., "Investigating Violence."

21. Women in Global Health, "Her Stories: Ending Sexual Exploitation, Abuse and Harassment of Women Health Workers" (Women in Global Health, December 2022), https://

womeningh.org/wp-content/uploads/2023/02/HealthToo-Policy-Report.pdf; L. T. Marufu, "Barriers and Facilitators of Female Community Health Workers When Performing Their Roles: A Study in Ssisa Sub County, Wakiso District, Uganda," *BMC Proceedings* 11, Suppl 6 (2017): 10, 24–25; Closser et al., "Breaking the Silence"; J Dasgupta et al., "The Safety of Women Health Workers at the Frontlines," *Indian Journal of Medical Ethics* 2, no. 3 (September 2017); Zubia Mumtaz et al., "Gender-Based Barriers to Primary Health Care Provision in Pakistan: The Experience of Female Providers," *Health Policy and Planning* 18, no. 3 (September 1, 2003): 261–69; Emilija Zabiliūtė, "Claiming Status and Contesting Sexual Violence and Harassment among Community Health Activists in Delhi," *Gender, Place & Culture* 27, no. 1 (2020): 52–68; Sharmila Devi, "COVID-19 Exacerbates Violence against Health Workers," *The Lancet* 396, no. 10252 (September 5, 2020): 658.

22. World Health Organization, "Delivered by Women"; Closser et al., "Breaking the Silence"; International Labour Organization, "Safe and Healthy Working Environments Free from Violence and Harassment" (ILO, 2020).

23. George et al., "Violence against Female"; Closser et al., "Breaking the Silence"; International Labour Organization, "Safe and Healthy Working Environments."

24. National Health Mission, "Mobilizing for Action on Violence Against Women: A Hand Book for ASHA" (National Health Mission, 2016); National Rural Health Mission, "Guidelines for Community Processes" (National Rural Health Mission, 2013); C. K. Mishra, "Safety Measures for ASHAs," National Health Systems Resource Centre, Jan. 29, 2016, https://nhsrcindia.org/sites/default/files/2021-03/Safety%20measures%20for%20ASHAs_29.01.2016.pdf.

25. International Labour Organization, "Safe and Healthy Working Environments"; Closser et al., "Breaking the Silence."

26. Sarah Ahmed, "'I Am My Own Person,' Women's Agency Inside and Outside the Home in Rural Pakistan," *Gender, Place & Culture* 27, no. 8 (August 2, 2020): 1176–94; Closser, "Pakistan's Lady Health Worker."

27. Morgana G. Martins Krieger et al., "How Do Community Health Workers Institutionalise: An Analysis of Brazil's CHW Programme," *Global Public Health* 17, no. 8 (August 3, 2022): 1507–24; Terry Mason et al., "Winning Policy Change to Promote Community Health Workers: Lessons From Massachusetts in the Health Reform Era," *American Journal of Public Health* 101, no. 12 (December 2011): 2211–16.

28. World Health Organization, "WHO Guideline on Health Policy."

29. Schaaf et al., "Report on the 'Think-in.'"

30. Martin Oliver et al., "What Do Community Health Workers Have to Say about Their Work, and How Can This Inform Improved Programme Design? A Case Study with CHWs within Kenya," *Global Health Action* 8 (2015): 27168; Abigail H. Neel et al., "30 Years of Polio Campaigns in Ethiopia, India and Nigeria: The Impacts of Campaign Design on Vaccine Hesitancy and Health Worker Motivation," *BMJ Global Health* 6, no. 8 (August 1, 2021): e006002.

BIBLIOGRAPHY

Adams, Vincanne. *Metrics: What Counts in Global Health*. Duke University Press, 2016.

Agarwala, Rina. "Reshaping the Social Contract: Emerging Relations between the State and Informal Labor in India." *Theory and Society* 37, no. 4 (August 1, 2008): 375–408. https://doi.org/10.1007/s11186-008-9061-5.

Ahmed, Sarah. "'I Am My Own Person,' Women's Agency inside and Outside the Home in Rural Pakistan." *Gender, Place & Culture* 27, no. 8 (August 2, 2020): 1176–94. https://doi.org/10.1080/0966369X.2019.1664420.

Akintola, Olagoke. "Unpaid HIV/AIDS–Care in Southern Africa: Forms, Context, and Implications." *Feminist Economics* 14, no. 4 (2008): 117. https://doi.org/10.1080/13545700802263004.

Arole, Mabelle, and Rajanikant Arole. "A Comprehensive Rural Health Project in Jamkhed (India)." In *Health for the People*, edited by Kenneth W. Newell. World Health Organization, 1975.

Arole, Mabelle, and Rajanikant Arole. *Jamkhed: A Comprehensive Rural Health Project*. Macmillan, 1994.

Asthana, Sumegha, and Kaveri Mayra. "India's One Million Accredited Social Health Activists (ASHA) Win the Global Health Leaders Award at the 75th World Health Assembly: Time to Move beyond Rhetoric to Action?" *The Lancet Regional Health – Southeast Asia* 3 (August 1, 2022). https://doi.org/10.1016/j.lansea.2022.100029.

Banerji, Debabar. "Politics of Rural Health in India." *International Journal of Health Services* 35, no. 4 (October 1, 2005): 783–96. https://doi.org/10.2190/1G7Y-KVE3-B6YV-ANE9.

Bellacasa, María Puig de la. "'Nothing Comes Without Its World': Thinking with Care." *Sociological Review* 60, no. 2 (2012): 197–216. https://doi.org/10.1111/j.1467-954X.2012.02070.x.

Besky, Sarah. "Can a Plantation Be Fair? Paradoxes and Possibilities in Fair Trade Darjeeling Tea Certification." *Anthropology of Work Review* 29, no. 1 (2008): 1–9. https://doi.org/10.1111/j.1548-1417.2008.00006.x.

Bhatia, Kavita. "Community Health Worker Programs in India: A Rights-Based Review." *Perspectives in Public Health* 134, no. 5 (2014): 276–82. https://doi.org/10.1177/1757913914543446.

Bhatia, Kavita. "Performance-Based Incentives of the ASHA Scheme: Stakeholders' Perspectives." *Economic and Political Weekly* 49, no. 22 (2014): 145–51. http://www.jstor.org/stable/24479649.

Biehl, João. "Theorizing Global Health." *Medicine Anthropology Theory* 3, no. 2 (September 13, 2016). https://doi.org/10.17157/mat.3.2.434.

Biruk, Cal (Crystal). "Capture-Recapture." *American Ethnologist* 49, no. 4 (2022): 549–62. https://doi.org/10.1111/amet.13107.

Bose, Ashish. *Studies in Social Dynamics of Primary Health Care*. Hindustan Publishing Corporation (India), 1983.

Bowser, Diana, Adeyemi Okunogbe, Elizabeth Oliveras, Laura Subramanian, and Tyler Morrill. "A Cost-Effectiveness Analysis of Community Health Workers in Mozambique." *Journal of Primary Care & Community Health* 6, no. 4 (October 1, 2015): 227–32. https://doi.org/10.1177/2150131915579653.

Brown, Hannah, and Ruth J. Prince. "Introduction: Volunteer Labor—Pasts and Futures of Work, Development, and Citizenship in East Africa." *African Studies Review* 58, no. 2 (September 2015): 29–42. https://doi.org/10.1017/asr.2015.36.

Campbell, C., and K. Scott. "Retreat from Alma Ata? The WHO's Report on Task Shifting to Community Health Workers for AIDS Care in Poor Countries." *Global Public Health* 6, no. 2 (March 1, 2011): 125–38. https://doi.org/10.1080/17441690903334232.

Chant, Sylvia. "The 'Feminisation of Poverty' and the 'Feminisation' of Anti-Poverty Programmes: Room for Revision?" *Journal of Development Studies* 44, no. 2 (February 2008): 165–97.

Chant, Sylvia. "Women, Girls and World Poverty: Empowerment, Equality or Essentialism?" *International Development Planning Review* 38, no. 1 (2016): 1–24.

Ciotti, Manuela. "At the Margins of Feminist Politics? A Comparative Analysis of Women in Dalit Politics and Hindu Right Organisations in Northern India." *Contemporary South Asia* 15, no. 4 (December 1, 2006): 437–52. https://doi.org/10.1080/09584930701330022.

Closser, Svea. *Chasing Polio in Pakistan: Why the World's Largest Public Health Initiative May Fail*. Vanderbilt University Press, 2010.

Closser, Svea. "'I Need Money, That's the Only Reason I Do It': Youth 'Volunteers,' Unemployment, and International Action in Pakistan's Health Sector." In *The Crisis in Global Youth Unemployment*, edited by T. Mayer, Sujata Moorti, and Jamie McCallum. Routledge, 2018.

Closser, Svea. "Pakistan's Lady Health Worker Labor Movement and the Moral Economy of Heroism." *Annals of Anthropological Practice* 39, no. 1 (May 1, 2015): 16–28. https://doi.org/10.1111/napa.12061.

Closser, Svea. "The Corruption Game: Health Systems, International Agencies, and the State in South Asia." *Medical Anthropology Quarterly* 34, no. 2 (2020): 268–85. https://doi.org/10.1111/maq.12549.

Closser, Svea, and Rashid Jooma. "Why We Must Provide Better Support for Pakistan's Female Frontline Health Workers." *PLoS Med* 10, no. 10 (October 8, 2013): e1001528. https://doi.org/10.1371/journal.pmed.1001528.

Closser, Svea, Kenneth Maes, Erick Gong, Neha Sharma, Yihenew Tesfaye, Roza Abesha, Mikayla Hyman, Natalie Meyer, and Jeffrey Carpenter. "Political Connections and Psychosocial Wellbeing among Women's Development Army Leaders in Rural Amhara, Ethiopia: Towards a Holistic Understanding of Community Health Workers' Socioeconomic Status." *Social Science & Medicine* 266 (December 1, 2020): 113373. https://doi.org/10.1016/j.socscimed.2020.113373.

Closser, Svea, Emily Mendenhall, Peter Brown, Rachel Neill, and Judith Justice. "The Anthropology of Health Systems: A History and Review." In "Health systems performance or performing health systems?," special issue of *Social Science & Medicine* 300 (May 1, 2022): 114314. https://doi.org/10.1016/j.socscimed.2021.114314.

Closser, Svea, Harriet Napier, Kenneth Maes, Roza Abesha, Hana Gebremariam, Grace Backe, Sarah Fossett, and Yihenew Tesfaye. "Does Volunteer Community Health Work Empower Women? Evidence from Ethiopia's Women's Development Army." *Health Policy and Planning* 34, no. 4 (May 1, 2019): 298–306. https://doi.org/10.1093/heapol/czz025.

Closser, Svea, Anat Rosenthal, Judith Justice, Kenneth Maes, Marium Sultan, Sarah Banerji, Hailom Banteyerga Amaha, Ranjani Gopinath, Patricia Omidian, and Laetitia Nyirazinyoye. "Per Diems in Polio Eradication: Perspectives From Community Health Workers and Officials." *American Journal of Public Health* 107, no. 9 (September 2017): 1470–76. https://doi.org/10.2105/AJPH.2017.303886.

Closser, Svea, Marium Sultan, Roosa Tikkanen, Shalini Singh, Arman Majidulla, Kenneth Maes, Sue Gerber, et al. "Breaking the Silence on Gendered Harassment and Assault of Community Health Workers: An Analysis of Ethnographic Studies." *BMJ Global Health* 8, no. 5 (May 1, 2023): e011749. https://doi.org/10.1136/bmjgh-2023-011749.

Colvin, Christopher J., and Alison Swartz. "Extension Agents or Agents of Change?" *Annals of Anthropological Practice* 39, no. 1 (May 1, 2015): 29–41. https://doi.org/10.1111/napa.12062.

Committee on Empowerment of Women (2010–2011), Fifteenth Lok Sabha. "Eleventh Report: Working Conditions of ASHAs." Lok Sabha Secretariat, September 2011.

Cooper, Amy. "What Does Health Activism Mean in Venezuela's Barrio Adentro Program? Understanding Community Health Work in Political and Cultural Context." *Annals of Anthropological Practice* 39, no. 1 (2015): 58–72. https://doi.org/10.1111/napa.12063.

Cueto, M. "The Origins of Primary Health Care and Selective Primary Health Care." *American Journal of Public Health* 94, no. 11 (November 1, 2004): 1864–74.

Dasgupta, J., J. Velankar, P. Borah, and G. Nath. "The Safety of Women Health Workers at the Frontlines." *Indian Journal of Medical Ethics* 2, no. 3 (September 2017). https://doi.org/10.20529/IJME.2017.043.

Dasgupta, Jashodhara, and Kanika Jha Kingra. "Women Workers at the Forefront of COVID-19: A Roadmap for Recovery and Resilience in India." In *The Political Economy of Post-COVID Life and Work in the Global South: Pandemic and Precarity*, edited by Sandya Hewamanne and Smytta Yadav. International Political Economy Series. Springer International Publishing, 2022. https://doi.org/10.1007/978-3-030-93228-2_6.

Davala, Sarath. "Independent Trade Unionism in West Bengal." *Economic and Political Weekly* 31, no. 52 (1996): L44–49. http://www.jstor.org/stable/4404934.

Devi, Sharmila. "COVID-19 Exacerbates Violence against Health Workers." *The Lancet* 396, no. 10252 (September 5, 2020): 658. https://doi.org/10.1016/S0140-6736(20)31858-4.

Donner, Henrike. "'The Girls Are Alright': Beauty Work and Neoliberal Regimes of Responsibility among Young Women in Urban India." *Critique of Anthropology* 43, no. 4 (December 1, 2023): 399–421. https://doi.org/10.1177/0308275X231216255.

Duclos, Diane, Sylvain L. Faye, Tidiane Ndoye, and Loveday Penn-Kekana. "Envisioning, Evaluating and Co-Enacting Performance in Global Health Interventions: Ethnographic Insights from Senegal." *Anthropology in Action* 26, no. 1 (2019): 21–30. https://doi.org/10.3167/aia.2019.260103.

Erikson, S. "Global Health Business: The Production and Performativity of Statistics in Sierra Leone and Germany." *Medical Anthropology* 31, no. 4 (2012): 367–84.

Fan, Elsa L. "Counting Results: Performance-Based Financing and HIV Testing among MSM in China." *Critical Public Health* 27, no. 2 (March 15, 2017): 217–27. https://doi.org/10.1080/09581596.2016.1259458.

Fan, Elsa, and Elanah Uretsky. "In Search of Results: Anthropological Interrogations of Evidence-Based Global Health." *Critical Public Health* 27, no. 2 (2017): 157–62.

Farmer, Paul, Arthur Kleinman, Jim Kim, and Matthew Basilico. *Reimagining Global Health: An Introduction*. University of California Press, 2013.

Fernandes, Leela. "Culture, Structure and Working Class Politics." *Economic and Political Weekly* 33, no. 52 (1998): L53–60. http://www.jstor.org/stable/4407516.

Frankfurter, Raphael. "Conjuring Biosecurity in the Post-Ebola Kissi Triangle: The Magic of Paperwork in a Frontier Clinic." *Medical Anthropology Quarterly* 33, no. 4 (2019): 517–38. https://doi.org/10.1111/maq.12528.

Friedemann-Sánchez, Greta, and Joan M. Griffin. "Defining the Boundaries between Unpaid Labor and Unpaid Caregiving: Review of the Social and Health Sciences Literature." *Journal of Human Development and Capabilities* 12, no. 4 (November 1, 2011): 511–34. https://doi.org/10.1080/19452829.2011.613370.

Garg, Samir, and Suchi Pande. "Learning to Sustain Change: Mitanin Community Health Workers Promote Public Accountability in India." Accountability Research Center, August 2018.

George, Asha S., Frances E. McConville, Shaheem de Vries, Gustavo Nigenda, Shabnum Sarfraz, and Michelle McIsaac. "Violence against Female Health Workers Is Tip of Iceberg of Gender Power Imbalances." *BMJ* 371 (October 27, 2020): m3546. https://doi.org/10.1136/bmj.m3546.

Gimbel, Sarah, Baltazar Chilundo, Nora Kenworthy, Celso Inguane, David Citrin, Rachel Chapman, Kenneth Sherr, and James Pfeiffer. "Donor Data Vacuuming." *Medicine Anthropology Theory* 5, no. 2 (May 15, 2018). https://doi.org/10.17157/mat.5.2.537.

Glenton, Claire, Inger B. Scheel, Sabina Pradhan, Simon Lewin, Stephen Hodgins, and Vijaya Shrestha. "The Female Community Health Volunteer Programme in Nepal: Decision Makers' Perceptions of Volunteerism, Payment and Other Incentives." *Social Science & Medicine* 70, no. 12 (June 2010): 1920–27. https://doi.org/10.1016/j.socscimed.2010.02.034.

Gold, Ann. "New Light in the House: Schooling Girls in Rural North India." In *Everyday Life in South Asia*, edited by Diane Mines and Sarah Lamb. Indiana University Press, 2002.

Gold, Ann. "Purdah Is as Purdah's Kept." In *Listen to the Heron's Words*, edited by Gloria Raheja and Ann Gold. University of California Press, 1994.

Gold, Ann Grodzins, and Bhoju Ram Gujar. *In the Time of Trees and Sorrows: Nature, Power, and Memory in Rajasthan*. Duke University Press, 2002.

Gupta, Akhil. *Red Tape: Bureaucracy, Structural Violence, and Poverty in India*. Duke University Press, 2012.

Haines, Andy, David Sanders, Uta Lehmann, Alexander K. Rowe, Joy E. Lawn, Steve Jan, Damian G. Walker, and Zulfiqar Bhutta. "Achieving Child Survival Goals: Potential Contribution of Community Health Workers." *The Lancet* 369, no. 9579 (2007): 2121–31. https://doi.org/10.1016/S0140-6736(07)60325-0.

Hanefeld, J., and M. Musheke. "What Impact Do Global Health Initiatives Have on Human Resources for Antiretroviral Treatment Roll-out? A Qualitative Policy Analysis of Implementation Processes in Zambia." *Human Resources for Health* 7, no. 8 (2009).

Holmström, Mark. *Industry and Inequality: The Social Anthropology of Indian Labour*. Cambridge University Press, 1984.

Hutchinson, Eleanor, Susan Nayiga, Christine Nabirye, Lilian Taaka, and Sarah G. Staedke. "Data Value and Care Value in the Practice of Health Systems: A Case Study in Uganda." *Social Science & Medicine* 211 (August 1, 2018): 123–30. https://doi.org/10.1016/j.socscimed.2018.05.039.

International Labour Organization. "Safe and Healthy Working Environments Free from Violence and Harassment." ILO, 2020.

Jeffery, Patricia, and Roger Jeffery. "Killing My Heart's Desire: Education and Female Autonomy in Rural North India." In *Women as Subjects: South Asian Histories*, edited by Nita Kumar, 125–71. University Press of Virginia, 1994.

Joshi, Sujay R., and Matthew George. "Healthcare through Community Participation: Role of ASHAs." *Economic and Political Weekly* 47, no. 10 (2012): 70–76. http://www.jstor.org/stable/41419935.

Justice, Judith. "Can Socio-Cultural Information Improve Health Planning? A Case Study of Nepal's Assistant Nurse-Midwife." *Social Science & Medicine* 19, no. 3 (1984): 193–98. https://doi.org/10.1016/0277-9536(84)90210-7.

Justice, Judith. *Policies, Plans, and People.* University of California Press, 1986.

Kalbarczyk, Anna, Svea Closser, Selamawit Hirpa, Utsamani Cintyamena, Lutfhi Azizatun-nisa, Priyanka Agrawal, Ahmad Omid Rahimi, et al. "A Light Touch Intervention with a Heavy Lift—Gender, Space and Risk in a Global Vaccination Programme." *Global Public Health* 17, no. 12 (July 18, 2022): 1–14. https://doi.org/10.1080/17441692.2022.2099930.

Kalofonos, Ippolytos. "'All They Do Is Pray': Community Labour and the Narrowing of 'Care' during Mozambique's HIV Scale-Up." *Global Public Health* 9, no. 1–2 (February 12, 2014): 7–24. https://doi.org/10.1080/17441692.2014.881527.

Karim, Lamia. "NGOs, State and Neoliberal Development in South Asia: The Paradigmatic Case of Bangladesh in a Global Perspective." In *Routledge Handbook of Gender in South Asia*, 289–302. Routledge, 2021. https://www.taylorfrancis.com/chapters/edit/10.4324/9781003043102-25/ngos-state-neoliberal-development-south-asia-lamia-karim.

Keshavjee, M. D. Salmaan. *Blind Spot: How Neoliberalism Infiltrated Global Health.* University of California Press, 2014.

Kielmann, Karina. "The Ethnographic Lens." In *Health Policy and Systems Research: A Methodology Reader*, edited by Lucy Gilson. World Health Organization, 2012.

Kim, J. Y., J. V. Millen, A. Irwin, and E. Gershman, eds. *Dying for Growth: Global Inequality and the Health of the Poor.* Common Courage Press, 2002.

Kingori, Patricia, and René Gerrets. "Morals, Morale and Motivations in Data Fabrication: Medical Research Fieldworkers Views and Practices in Two Sub-Saharan African Contexts." *Social Science & Medicine* 166 (October 1, 2016): 150–59. https://doi.org/10.1016/j.socscimed.2016.08.019.

Kingori, Patricia, and René Gerrets. "The Masking and Making of Fieldworkers and Data in Postcolonial Global Health Research Contexts." *Critical Public Health* 29, no. 4 (August 8, 2019): 494–507. https://doi.org/10.1080/09581596.2019.1609650.

Kingori, Patricia, Francis Kombe, and Alexandra Fehr. "Making Global Health 'Work': Frontline Workers' Labour in Research and Interventions." *Global Public Health* 17, no. 12 (December 2, 2022): 4077–86. https://doi.org/10.1080/17441692.2022.2139852.

Kleinman, Arthur. "Four Social Theories for Global Health." *Lancet* 375, no. 9725 (2010): 1518–19.

Krieger, Morgana G. Martins, Clare Wenham, Denise Nacif Pimenta, Theresia E. Nkya, Brunah Schall, Ana Carolina Nunes, Ana De Menezes, and Gabriela Lotta. "How Do Community Health Workers Institutionalise: An Analysis of Brazil's CHW Programme." *Global Public Health* 17, no. 8 (August 3, 2022): 1507–24. https://doi.org/10.1080/17441692.2021.1940236.

Leslie, Charles. "What Caused India's Massive Community Health Workers Scheme: A Sociology of Knowledge." *Social Science & Medicine* 21, no. 8 (January 1, 1985): 923–30. https://doi.org/10.1016/0277-9536(85)90150-9.

Livingston, Julie. *Improvising Medicine: An African Oncology Ward in an Emerging Cancer Epidemic.* Duke University Press, 2012.

Lock, Margaret, and Vinh-Kim Nguyen. *An Anthropology of Biomedicine.* John Wiley & Sons, 2011.

Logan, Ryan I. "'A Poverty in Understanding': Assessing the Structural Challenges Experienced by Community Health Workers and Their Clients." *Global Public Health* 15, no. 1 (January 2, 2020): 137–50. https://doi.org/10.1080/17441692.2019.1656275.

Lorway, Robert. "Making Global Health Knowledge: Documents, Standards, and Evidentiary Sovereignty in HIV Interventions in South India." *Critical Public Health* 27, no. 2 (March 15, 2017): 177–92. https://doi.org/10.1080/09581596.2016.1262941.

Maes, Kenneth. "Community Health Workers and Social Change:" *Annals of Anthropological Practice* 39, no. 1 (May 1, 2015): 1–15. https://doi.org/10.1111/napa.12060.

Maes, Kenneth. *The Lives of Community Health Workers: Local Labor and Global Health in Urban Ethiopia*. Routledge, 2016.

Maes, Kenneth. "Volunteerism or Labor Exploitation? Harnessing the Volunteer Spirit to Sustain AIDS Treatment Programs in Urban Ethiopia." *Human Organization* 71, no. 1 (January 1, 2012): 54–64. http://www.metapress.com/content/AXM39467485M22W4.

Maes, Kenneth. "'Volunteers Are Not Paid Because They Are Priceless': Community Health Worker Capacities and Values in an AIDS Treatment Intervention in Urban Ethiopia." *Medical Anthropology Quarterly* 29, no. 1 (2015): 97–115. https://doi.org/10.1111/maq.12136.

Maes, Kenneth C., Brandon A. Kohrt, and Svea Closser. "Culture, Status and Context in Community Health Worker Pay: Pitfalls and Opportunities for Policy Research. A Commentary on Glenton et al. (2010)." *Social Science & Medicine* 71, no. 8 (October 2010): 1375–78. https://doi.org/10.1016/j.socscimed.2010.06.020.

Maes, Kenneth, Svea Closser, and Ippolytos Kalofonos. "Listening to Community Health Workers: How Ethnographic Research Can Inform Positive Relationships Among Community Health Workers, Health Institutions, and Communities." *American Journal of Public Health* 104, no. 5 (May 2014): e5–9. https://doi.org/10.2105/AJPH.2014.301907.

Maes, Kenneth, Svea Closser, Yihenew Tesfaye, and Roza Abesha. "Psychosocial Distress among Unpaid Community Health Workers in Rural Ethiopia: Comparing Leaders in Ethiopia's Women's Development Army to Their Peers." *Social Science & Medicine* 230 (June 1, 2019): 138–46. https://doi.org/10.1016/j.socscimed.2019.04.005.

Maes, Kenneth, Svea Closser, Ethan Vorel, and Yihenew Tesfaye. "Using Community Health Workers." *Annals of Anthropological Practice* 39, no. 1 (May 1, 2015): 42–57. https://doi.org/10.1111/napa.12064.

Maes, Kenneth, and Ippolytos Kalofonos. "Becoming and Remaining Community Health Workers: Perspectives from Ethiopia and Mozambique." *Social Science & Medicine* 87 (June 1, 2013): 52–59. https://doi.org/10.1016/j.socscimed.2013.03.026.

Maru, Rushikesh. "Community Health Worker: Some Aspects of the Experience at the National Level." *Medico Friend Circle Bulletin*, March 1980, 1–5.

Marufu, L. T. "Barriers and Facilitators of Female Community Health Workers when Performing Their Roles: A Study in Ssisa Sub County, Wakiso District, Uganda." *BMC Proceedings* 11, Suppl 6 (2017): 10, 24–25.

Mason, Katherine. *Infectious Change*. Stanford University Press, 2016.

Mason, Terry, Geoffrey W. Wilkinson, Angela Nannini, Cindy Marti Martin, Durrell J. Fox, and Gail Hirsch. "Winning Policy Change to Promote Community Health Workers: Lessons From Massachusetts in The Health Reform Era." *American Journal of Public Health* 101, no. 12 (December 2011): 2211–16. https://doi.org/10.2105/AJPH.2011.300402.

Maupin, Jonathan N. "Shifting Identities:" *Annals of Anthropological Practice* 39, no. 1 (2015): 73–88. https://doi.org/10.1111/napa.12065.

McKay, Ramah. "Global Health's Durable Dreams: Ethnography, 'Community Health Workers' and Health without Health Infrastructure." *Africa* 90, no. 1 (January 2020): 95–111. https://doi.org/10.1017/S0001972019000950.

Mies, Maria. "Dynamics of Sexual Division of Labour and Capital Accumulation: Women Lace Workers of Narsapur." *Economic and Political Weekly* 16, no. 10/12 (March 1981): 487–500.

Mishra, Arima. "'Trust and Teamwork Matter': Community Health Workers' Experiences in Integrated Service Delivery in India." *Global Public Health* 9, no. 8 (September 14, 2014): 960–74. https://doi.org/10.1080/17441692.2014.934877.

Mishra, C. K. "Safety Measures for ASHAs." National Health Systems Resource Centre, Jan. 29, 2016. https://nhsrcindia.org/sites/default/files/2021-03/Safety%20measures%20for%20ASHAs_29.01.2016.pdf.

Molyneux, Maxine. "Mothers at the Service of the New Poverty Agenda: Progresa/Oportunidades, Mexico's Conditional Transfer Programme." *Social Policy & Administration* 40, no. 4 (2006): 425–49. https://doi.org/10.1111/j.1467-9515.2006.00497.x.

Morgan, Lynn M. *Community Participation in Health: The Politics of Primary Care in Costa Rica.* Cambridge University Press, 1993.

Mumtaz, Zubia, Sarah Salway, Muneeba Waseem, and Nighat Umer. "Gender-Based Barriers to Primary Health Care Provision in Pakistan: The Experience of Female Providers." *Health Policy and Planning* 18, no. 3 (September 1, 2003): 261–69. https://doi.org/10.1093/heapol/czg032.

Murphy, Michelle. "The Girl: Mergers of Feminism and Finance in Neoliberal Times." *The Scholar & Feminist Online* 11, no. 1-2 (July 8, 2013). https://sfonline.barnard.edu/the-girl-mergers-of-feminism-and-finance-in-neoliberal-times.

Nading, Alex M. "Dengue Mosquitoes Are Single Mothers: Biopolitics Meets Ecological Aesthetics in Nicaraguan Community Health Work." *Cultural Anthropology* 27, no. 4 (2012): 572–96. https://doi.org/10.1111/j.1548-1360.2012.01162.x.

Nading, Alex M. "'Love Isn't There in Your Stomach.'" *Medical Anthropology Quarterly* 27, no. 1 (2013): 84–102. https://doi.org/10.1111/maq.12017.

Nandi, Sulakshana, and Helen Schneider. "Addressing the Social Determinants of Health: A Case Study from the Mitanin (Community Health Worker) Programme in India." *Health Policy and Planning* 29, no. suppl. 2 (September 1, 2014): ii71–81. https://doi.org/10.1093/heapol/czu074.

National Health Mission. "Mobilizing for Action on Violence Against Women: A Hand Book for ASHA." National Health Mission, 2016.

National Rural Health Mission. "Guidelines for Community Processes." National Rural Health Mission, 2013.

Neel, Abigail H., Svea Closser, Catherine Villanueva, Piyusha Majumdar, S. D. Gupta, Daniel Krugman, Oluwaseun Oladapo Akinyemi, Wakgari Deressa, Anna Kalbarczyk, and Olakunle Alonge. "30 Years of Polio Campaigns in Ethiopia, India and Nigeria: The Impacts of Campaign Design on Vaccine Hesitancy and Health Worker Motivation." *BMJ Global Health* 6, no. 8 (August 1, 2021): e006002. https://doi.org/10.1136/bmjgh-2021-006002.

Neve, Geert de. "'Keeping It in the Family': Work, Education and Gender Hierarchies among Tiruppur's Industrial Capitalists." In *Being Middle-Class in India.* Routledge, 2011.

Newell, Kenneth W. *Health by the People.* World Health Organization, 1975. https://apps.who.int/iris/handle/10665/40514.

Nichter, Mark A. "The Primary Health Center as a Social System: PHC, Social Status, and the Issue of Team-Work in South Asia." *Social Science & Medicine* 23, no. 4 (January 1, 1986): 347–55. https://doi.org/10.1016/0277-9536(86)90077-8.

Nielsen, Kenneth. "Women's Activism in the Singur Movement, West Bengal." In *Women, Gender and Everyday Social Transformation in India*, edited by Anne Waldrop and Kenneth Nielsen, 203–18. Anthem Press, 2014.

Nordfeldt, Cecilie, and Sidsel Roalkvam. "Choosing Vaccination: Negotiating Child Protec-tion and Good Citizenship in Modern India." *Forum for Development Studies* 37, no. 3 (November 1, 2010): 327–47. https://doi.org/10.1080/08039410.2010.513402.

Odendaal, Willem A., Jocelyn Anstey Watkins, Natalie Leon, Jane Goudge, Frances Griffiths, Mark Tomlinson, and Karen Daniels. "Health Workers' Perceptions and Experiences of Using mHealth Technologies to Deliver Primary Healthcare Services: A Qualitative Evidence Synthesis." *Cochrane Database of Systematic Reviews*, no. 3 (2020). https://doi.org/10.1002/14651858.CD011942.pub2.

Oliver, Martin, Anne Geniets, Niall Winters, Isabella Rega, and Simon M. Mbae. "What Do Community Health Workers Have to Say about Their Work, and How Can This Inform Improved Programme Design? A Case Study with CHWs within Kenya." *Global Health Action* 8 (2015): 27168. https://doi.org/10.3402/gha.v8.27168.

One Million Community Health Workers Campaign. "One Million Community Health Workers Map," 2018. http://1millionhealthworkers.org/operations-room-map.

"One Million Community Health Workers: Technical Task Force Report." Earth Institute at Columbia University, 2013. http://1millionhealthworkers.org/files/2013/01/1mCHW_TechnicalTaskForceReport.pdf.

Oni-Orisan, Adeola. "The Obligation to Count." In *Metrics*, edited by Vincanne Adams, 82–101. Duke University Press, 2016.

Osella, Filippo, and Caroline Osella. "From Transience to Immanence: Consumption, Life-Cycle and Social Mobility in Kerala, South India." *Modern Asian Studies* 33, no. 4 (October 1999): 989–1020. https://doi.org/10.1017/S0026749X99003479.

Palriwala, Rajni, and N. Neetha. "Care Arrangements and Bargains: Anganwadi and Paid Domestic Workers in India." *International Labour Review* 149, no. 4 (2010): 511–27. https://doi.org/10.1111/j.1564-913X.2010.00101.x.

Pande, Suchi. "Community Health Workers as Rights Defenders: The Mitanin Experience in India." *Development in Practice* 33, no 8 (2023): 939–44. https://doi.org/10.1080/09614524.2023.2213862.

Parry, Jonathan. "Company and Contract Labour in a Central Indian Steel Plant." *Economy and Society* 42, no. 3 (August 1, 2013): 348–74. https://doi.org/10.1080/03085147.2013.772761.

Perry, H. B., R. Zulliger, and M. M. Rogers. "Community Health Workers in Low-, Mid-dle-, and High-Income Countries: An Overview of Their History, Recent Evolution, and Current Effectiveness." *Annual Review of Public Health* 35 (2014): 399–421. https://doi.org/10.1146/Annurev-Publhealth-032013-182354.

Perry, Henry B., and Jon Rohde. "The Jamkhed Comprehensive Rural Health Project and the Alma-Ata Vision of Primary Health Care." *American Journal of Public Health* 109, no. 5 (March 21, 2019): 699–704. https://doi.org/10.2105/AJPH.2019.304968.

Pfeiffer, James. "International NGOs in the Mozambique Health Sector: The 'Velvet Glove' of Privatization." In *Unhealthy Health Policy*. AltaMira Press, 2004.

Pfeiffer, James, and Mark Nichter. "What Can Critical Medical Anthropology Contribute to Global Health?" *Medical Anthropology Quarterly* 22, no. 4 (December 2008): 410–15. https://doi.org/10.1111/j.1548-1387.2008.00041.x.

Prakash, Priyali. "Explained | All about India's ASHA Workers, Recipients of WHO's Global Leaders Award." *The Hindu*, May 28, 2022, sec. India. https://www.thehindu.com/news/national/explained-all-about-indias-asha-workers-recipients-of-whos-global-leaders-award/article65457663.ece.

Prince, Ruth, and Hannah Brown, eds. *Volunteer Economies: The Politics and Ethics of Volun-tary Labour in Africa*. James Currey, 2016.

Raheja, Gloria Goodwin, and Ann Grodzins Gold. *Listen to the Heron's Words: Reimagining Gender and Kinship in North India*. University of California Press, 1994.

Ramirez-Valles, Jesus. "Promoting Health, Promoting Women: The Construction of Female and Professional Identities in the Discourse of Community Health Workers." *Social Science & Medicine* 47, no. 11 (December 1998): 1749–62. https://doi.org/10.1016/S0277-9536(98)00246-9.

Rao, Lavanya, Ravi Prakash, Prathibha Rai, Mallika Tharakan, Kavitha DL, Arin Kar, Mohan HL, and Krishnamurthy Jayanna. "Investigating Violence against Accredited Social Health Activists (ASHAs): A Mixed Methods Study from Rural North Karnataka, India." *Journal of Global Health Reports* 5 (June 18, 2021): e2021054. https://doi.org/10.29392/001c.24351.

Ray, Panchali. "Women in/and Trade Unions: Consciousness, Agency, and (Im)Possibilities of Alliances amongst Nurses and Attendants in Kolkata." *Contemporary South Asia* 27, no. 4 (October 2, 2019): 502–15. https://doi.org/10.1080/09584935.2019.1667303.

Rifkin, Susan B. "Alma Ata after 40 Years: Primary Health Care and Health for All—from Consensus to Complexity." *BMJ Global Health* 3, suppl. 3 (December 1, 2018): e001188. https://doi.org/10.1136/bmjgh-2018-001188.

Roalkvam, Sidsel. "Health Governance in India: Citizenship as Situated Practice." *Global Public Health* 9, no. 8 (2014): 910–26.

RoyChowdhury, Supriya. "Old Classes and New Spaces: Urban Poverty, Unorganised Labour and New Unions." *Economic and Political Weekly* 38, no. 50 (2003): 5277–84. http://www.jstor.org/stable/4414402.

Sanchez, Andrew. *Criminal Capital: Violence, Corruption and Class in Industrial India*. Routledge, 2016.

Sanchez, Andrew. "Questioning Success: Dispossession and the Criminal Entrepreneur in Urban India." *Critique of Anthropology* 32, no. 4 (December 1, 2012): 435–57. https://doi.org/10.1177/0308275X12456652.

Sanchez, Andrew, and Christian Strümpell. "Sons of Soil, Sons of Steel: Autochthony, Descent and the Class Concept in Industrial India." *Modern Asian Studies* 48, no. 5 (September 2014): 1276–301. https://doi.org/10.1017/S0026749X14000213.

Sawadogo, N. Hélène, Hamidou Sanou, Jeremy A. Greene, and Vincent Duclos. "Promises and Perils of Mobile Health in Burkina Faso." *The Lancet* 398, no. 10302 (August 28, 2021): 738–39. https://doi.org/10.1016/S0140-6736(21)01001-1.

Saxena, Kiran. "The Hindu Trade Union Movement in India: The Bharatiya Mazdoor Sangh." *Asian Survey* 33, no. 7 (1993): 685–96. https://doi.org/10.2307/2645356.

Schaaf, Marta, Caitlin Warthin, Amy Manning, and Stephanie Topp. "Report on the 'Think-in' on Community Health Worker Voice, Power, and Citizens' Right to Health." Accountability Research Center, January 2018.

Scott, James C. *Weapons of the Weak*. Yale University Press, 1985.

Scott, Kerry, Asha S. George, and Rajani R. Ved. "Taking Stock of 10 Years of Published Research on the ASHA Programme: Examining India's National Community Health Worker Programme from a Health Systems Perspective." *Health Research Policy and Systems* 17, no. 1 (March 25, 2019): 29. https://doi.org/10.1186/s12961-019-0427-0.

Scott, Kerry, and Shobhit Shanker. "Tying Their Hands? Institutional Obstacles to the Success of the ASHA Community Health Worker Programme in Rural North India." *AIDS Care* 22, suppl. 2 (2010): 1606–12. https://doi.org/10.1080/09540121.2010.507751.

Sen, Binayak. "Myth of the Mitanin: Political Constraints on Structural Reforms in Healthcare in Chhattisgarh." *Medico Friend Circle Bulletin* 311 (2005): 12–17.

Sharma, Aradhana. "Crossbreeding Institutions, Breeding Struggle: Women's Empowerment, Neoliberal Governmentality, and State (Re)Formation in India." *Cultural Anthropology* 21, no. 1 (2006): 60–95.

Sharma, Reetu, Premila Webster, and Sanghita Bhattacharyya. "Factors Affecting the
Performance of Community Health Workers in India: A Multi-Stakeholder Perspective."
Global Health Action 7 (October 13, 2014). https://doi.org/10.3402/gha.v7.25352.

Shiffman, Jeremy, and Yusra Ribhi Shawar. "Strengthening Accountability of the Global
Health Metrics Enterprise." *The Lancet* 395, no. 10234 (May 2, 2020): 1452–56. https://doi.
org/10.1016/S0140-6736(20)30416-5.

Storeng, Katerini T., and Arima Mishra. "Politics and Practices of Global Health: Critical
Ethnographies of Health Systems." *Global Public Health* 9, no. 8 (September 14, 2014):
858–64. https://doi.org/10.1080/17441692.2014.941901.

Sundararaman, T. "Universalisation of ICDS and Community Health Worker Programmes:
Lessons from Chhattisgarh." *Economic and Political Weekly* 41, no. 34 (2006): 3674–79.
http://www.jstor.org/stable/4418616.

Swaminathan, Padmini. "The Formal Creation of Informality, and Therefore, Gender Injustice: Illustrations from India's Social Sector." *Indian Journal of Labour Economics* 58
(2015): 23–42.

Swartz, Alison. "Legacy, Legitimacy, and Possibility." *Medical Anthropology Quarterly* 27,
no. 2 (2013): 139–54. https://doi.org/10.1111/maq.12020.

Swartz, Alison, and Christopher J. Colvin. "'It's in Our Veins': Caring Natures and Material Motivations of Community Health Workers in Contexts of Economic Marginalisation." *Critical
Public Health* 25, no. 2 (July 30, 2014): 1–14. https://doi.org/10.1080/09581596.2014.941281.

Tichenor, Marlee. "Data Performativity, Performing Health Work: Malaria and Labor in Senegal." *Medical Anthropology* 36, no. 5 (2017): 436–48. https://doi.org/10.1080/01459740.2017
.1316722.

Tikkanen, Roosa Sofia, Svea Closser, Justine Prince, Priyankar Chand, and Judith Justice.
"An Anthropological History of Nepal's Female Community Health Volunteer Program:
Gender, Policy, and Social Change." *International Journal for Equity in Health* 23, no. 1
(April 13, 2024): 70. https://doi.org/10.1186/s12939-024-02177-5.

Tollman, S. M. "The Pholela Health Centre—the Origins of Community-Oriented Primary
Health Care (COPC)." *South African Medical Journal* 84, no. 10 (1994): 653–58. https://www.
ajol.info/index.php/samj/article/view/149397.

Trafford, Zara, Alison Swartz, and Christopher J. Colvin. "'Contract to Volunteer': South
African Community Health Worker Mobilization for Better Labor Protection." *NEW
SOLUTIONS: A Journal of Environmental and Occupational Health Policy* 27, no. 4 (Febru-
ary 1, 2018): 648–66. https://doi.org/10.1177/1048291117739529.

Tronto, Joan C. *Caring Democracy: Markets, Equality, and Justice.* New York University
Press, 2013.

Uretsky, Elanah. "'We Can't Do That Here': Negotiating Evidence in HIV Prevention Campaigns in Southwest China." *Critical Public Health* 27, no. 2 (March 15, 2017): 205–16.
https://doi.org/10.1080/09581596.2016.1264571.

Uzwiak, Beth A., and Siobhan Curran. "Gendering the Burden of Care: Health Reform and
the Paradox of Community Participation in Western Belize." *Medical Anthropology Quarterly* 30, no. 1 (2016): 100–121. https://doi.org/10.1111/maq.12195.

van de Ruit, Catherine. "Unintended Consequences of Community Health Worker Programs in South Africa." *Qualitative Health Research* 29, no. 11 (September 1, 2019): 1535–
48. https://doi.org/10.1177/1049732319857059.

van de Ruit, Catherine, and Alexandra Breckenridge. "South African Community Health Workers' Pursuit of Occupational Security." *Gender, Work & Organization* 31, no. 4 (2022), 1560–81. https://doi.org/10.1111/gwao.12854.

Vaughan, Kelsey, Maryse C. Kok, Sophie Witter, and Marjolein Dieleman. "Costs and Cost-Effectiveness of Community Health Workers: Evidence from a Literature Review." *Human Resources for Health* 13, no. 1 (September 1, 2015): 71. https://doi.org/10.1186/s12960-015-0070-y.

Ved, R., K. Scott, G. Gupta, O. Ummer, S. Singh, A. Srivastava, and A. S. George. "How Are Gender Inequalities Facing India's One Million ASHAs Being Addressed? Policy Origins and Adaptations for the World's Largest All-Female Community Health Worker Programme." *Human Resources for Health* 17, no. 1 (January 8, 2019): 3. https://doi.org/10.1186/s12960-018-0338-0.

Walt, Gill, and Lucy Gilson. *Community Health Workers in National Programmes: Just Another Pair of Hands?* Open University Press, 1990.

Wendland, Claire. *A Heart for the Work: Journeys Through an African Medical School.* University of Chicago Press, 2010.

Werner, David. "The Village Health Worker: Lackey or Liberator?" *World Health Forum* 2, no. 1 (1981): 46–54.

Wintrup, James. "Health by the People, Again? The Lost Lessons of Alma-Ata in a Community Health Worker Programme in Zambia." In "Health for all? Pasts, Presents and Futures of Universal Health Care and Universal Health Coverage," special issue of *Social Science & Medicine* 319 (February 1, 2023): 115257. https://doi.org/10.1016/j.socscimed.2022.115257.

Women in Global Health. "Her Stories: Ending Sexual Exploitation, Abuse and Harassment of Women Health Workers." Women in Global Health, December 2022. https://womeningh.org/wp-content/uploads/2023/02/HealthToo-Policy-Report.pdf.

Women in Global Health. "Subsidizing Global Health: Women's Unpaid Work in Health Systems." Women in Global Health, 2022. https://womeningh.org/wp-content/uploads/2022/07/Pay-Women-Report-July-7-Release.pdf.

World Health Organization. "Declaration of Alma-Ata." In *International Conference on Primary Health Care.* Alma-Ata, USSR, 1978.

World Health Organization. "Delivered by Women, Led by Men: A Gender and Equity Analysis of the Global Health and Social Workforce." World Health Organization, 2019. http://www.who.int/hrh/resources/health-observer24/en/.

World Health Organization. "WHO Guideline on Health Policy and System Support to Optimize Community Health Worker Programmes." World Health Organization, 2018.

Zabiliūtė, Emilija. "Claiming Status and Contesting Sexual Violence and Harassment among Community Health Activists in Delhi." *Gender, Place & Culture* 27, no. 1 (2020): 52–68.

INDEX

www.ingramcontent.com/pod-product-compliance
Lightning Source LLC
Chambersburg PA
CBHW030335270326
41926CB00010B/1631